T0226533

Sports Cardiology

Editors

AARON BAGGISH
ANDRÉ LA GERCHE

CARDIOLOGY CLINICS

www.cardiology.theclinics.com

Consulting Editors
ROSARIO FREEMAN
JORDAN M. PRUTKIN
DAVID M. SHAVELLE
AUDREY H. WU

November 2016 • Volume 34 • Number 4

ELSEVIER

1600 John F. Kennedy Boulevard • Suite 1800 • Philadelphia, Pennsylvania, 19103-2899

http://www.theclinics.com

CARDIOLOGY CLINICS Volume 34, Number 4
November 2016 ISSN 0733-8651, ISBN-13: 978-0-323-47680-5

Editor: Lauren Boyle
Developmental Editor: Alison Swety

© 2016 Elsevier Inc. All rights reserved.

This periodical and the individual contributions contained in it are protected under copyright by Elsevier, and the following terms and conditions apply to their use:

Photocopying

Single photocopies of single articles may be made for personal use as allowed by national copyright laws. Permission of the Publisher and payment of a fee is required for all other photocopying, including multiple or systematic copying, copying for advertising or promotional purposes, resale, and all forms of document delivery. Special rates are available for educational institutions that wish to make photocopies for non-profit educational classroom use. For information on how to seek permission visit www.elsevier.com/permissions or call: (+44) 1865 843830 (UK)/(+1) 215 239 3804 (USA).

Derivative Works

Subscribers may reproduce tables of contents or prepare lists of articles including abstracts for internal circulation within their institutions. Permission of the Publisher is required for resale or distribution outside the institution. Permission of the Publisher is required for all other derivative works, including compilations and translations (please consult www.elsevier.com/permissions).

Electronic Storage or Usage

Permission of the Publisher is required to store or use electronically any material contained in this periodical, including any article or part of an article (please consult www.elsevier.com/permissions). Except as outlined above, no part of this publication may be reproduced, stored in a retrieval system or transmitted in any form or by any means, electronic, mechanical, photo-copying, recording or otherwise, without prior written permission of the Publisher.

Notice

No responsibility is assumed by the Publisher for any injury and/or damage to persons or property as a matter of products liability, negligence or otherwise, or from any use or operation of any methods, products, instructions or ideas contained in the material herein. Because of rapid advances in the medical sciences, in particular, independent verification of diagnoses and drug dosages should be made.

Although all advertising material is expected to conform to ethical (medical) standards, inclusion in this publication does not constitute a guarantee or endorsement of the quality or value of such product or of the claims made of it by its manufacturer.

Cardiology Clinics (ISSN 0733-8651) is published quarterly by Elsevier Inc., 360 Park Avenue South, New York, NY 10010-1710. Months of issue are February, May, August, and November. Business and Editorial Offices: 1600 John F. Kennedy Blvd., Ste. 1800, Philadelphia, PA 19103-2899. Customer Service Office: 3251 Riverport Lane, Maryland Heights, MO 63043. Periodicals post-age paid at New York, NY and additional mailing offices. Subscription prices are $320.00 per year for US individuals, $581.00 per year for US institutions, $100.00 per year for US students and residents, $390.00 per year for Canadian individuals, $729.00 per year for Canadian institutions, $455.00 per year for international individuals, $729.00 per year for international institutions and $220.00 per year for Canadian and international students/residents. To receive student/resident rate, orders must be accompanied by name of affiliated institution, data of term, and the *signature* of program/residency coordinator on institution letterhead. Orders will be billed at individual rate until proof of status is received. Foreign air speed delivery is included in all *Clinics* subscription prices. All prices are subject to change without notice. **POSTMASTER:** Send address changes to *Cardiology Clinics*, Elsevier Health Sciences Division, Subscription Customer Service, 3251 Riverport Lane, Maryland Heights, MO 63043. **Customer Service: 1-800-654-2452 (U.S. and Canada); 314-447-8871 (outside U.S. and Canada). Fax: 314-447-8029. E-mail: journalscustomerservice-usa@ elsevier.com (for print support); journalsonlinesupport-usa@elsevier.com (for online support).**

Reprints. For copies of 100 or more, of articles in this publication, please contact the Commercial Reprints Department, Elsevier Inc., 360 Park Avenue South, New York, NY 10010-1710. Tel.: 212-633-3874; Fax: 212-633-3820; E-mail: reprints@elsevier.com.

Cardiology Clinics is also published in Spanish by McGraw-Hill Interamericana Editores S. A., P.O. Box 5-237, 06500, Mexico D. F., Mexico; in Portuguese by Reichmann and Alfonso Editores Rio de Janeiro, Brazil; and in Greek by Dimitrios P. Lagos, 8 Pondon Street, GR115-28 Ilissia, Greece.

Cardiology Clinics is covered in *MEDLINE/PubMed (Index Medicus), Excerpta Medica, The Cumulative Index to Nursing and Allied Health Literature (CINAHL).*

Contributors

EDITORIAL BOARD

ROSARIO FREEMAN, MD, MS, FACC
Associate Professor of Medicine; Director,
Coronary Care Unit; Director,
Echocardiography Laboratory, University of
Washington Medical Center, Seattle,
Washington

JORDAN M. PRUTKIN, MD, MHS, FHRS
Assistant Professor of Medicine, Division of
Cardiology/Electrophysiology, University of
Washington Medical Center, Seattle,
Washington

DAVID M. SHAVELLE, MD, FACC, FSCAI
Associate Professor, Keck School of Medicine;
Director, General Cardiovascular Fellowship
Program; Director, Cardiac Catheterization
Laboratory, Los Angeles County + USC
Medical Center; Division of Cardiovascular
Medicine, University of Southern California,
Los Angeles, California

AUDREY H. WU, MD
Assistant Professor, Internal Medicine,
University of Michigan, Ann Arbor,
Michigan

EDITORS

AARON BAGGISH, MD, FACC, FACSM
Director, Cardiovascular Performance
Program, Division of Cardiology,
Massachusetts General Hospital, Boston,
Massachusetts

ANDRÉ LA GERCHE, MBBS, PhD, FRACP, FESC
Associate Professor, Head, Department of
Sports Cardiology, Baker IDI Heart and
Diabetes Institute; Department of Cardiology,
Alfred Hospital, Melbourne, Victoria, Australia

AUTHORS

AARON BAGGISH, MD, FACC, FACSM
Director, Cardiovascular Performance
Program, Division of Cardiology,
Massachusetts General Hospital, Boston,
Massachusetts

ROBERT W. BATTLE, MD
Professor of Medicine and Pediatrics, Division
of Pediatric Cardiology, Department of
Pediatrics; Division of Cardiology, Department
of Internal Medicine, University of Virginia,
Charlottesville, Virginia

RHYS BEAUDRY, BSc
Department of Sports Cardiology, Baker IDI
Heart and Diabetes Institute, Melbourne,
Victoria, Australia; College of Nursing and
Health Innovation, University of Texas at
Arlington, Arlington, Texas

BIANCA C. BERNARDO, PhD
Baker IDI Heart and Diabetes Institute, Cardiac
Hypertrophy Laboratory, Melbourne, Victoria,
Australia

EDUARDO BOSSONE, MD
Professor, Department of Cardiology and
Cardiac Surgery, University Hospital San
Giovanni di Dio e Ruggi d'Aragona, Salerno, Italy

RAFFAELE CALABRÒ, MD
Professor, Department of Cardiology, Monaldi
Hospital, Chair of Cardiology, Second
University of Naples, Naples, Italy

ANTONELLO D'ANDREA, MD, PhD
Department of Cardiology, Monaldi Hospital,
Chair of Cardiology, Second University of
Naples, Naples, Italy

SHARLENE M. DAY, MD
Associate Professor of Internal Medicine,
Division of Cardiovascular Medicine,
Department of Internal Medicine, University of
Michigan School of Medicine, Ann Arbor,
Michigan

PETER N. DEAN, MD
Assistant Professor of Pediatrics, Division of
Pediatric Cardiology, Department of
Pediatrics, University of Virginia,
Charlottesville, Virginia

ADRIAN D. ELLIOTT, PhD
Centre for Heart Rhythm Disorders, South
Australian Health and Medical Research
Institute, Royal Adelaide Hospital, University of
Adelaide, Adelaide, South Australia, Australia

MAURIZIO GALDERISI, MD
Professor, Department of Advanced
Biomedical Sciences, Federico II University
Hospital, Naples, Italy

DAVID R. GOLDMANN, MD
Perelman School of Medicine, University of
Pennsylvania, Philadelphia,
Pennsylvania

MARK J. HAYKOWSKY, PhD, MSc
Department of Sports Cardiology, Baker IDI
Heart and Diabetes Institute, Melbourne,
Victoria, Australia; College of Nursing and
Health Innovation, University of Texas at
Arlington, Arlington, Texas

**ANDRÉ LA GERCHE, MBBS, PhD, FRACP,
FESC**
Associate Professor, Head, Department of
Sports Cardiology, Baker IDI Heart and
Diabetes Institute; Department of Cardiology,
Alfred Hospital, Melbourne, Victoria,
Australia

STEVEN LASCHER, DVM, PhD, MPH
Elsevier Clinical Solutions, Evidence-Based
Medicine Center, Philadelphia,
Pennsylvania

DENNIS H. LAU, MBBS, PhD
Centre for Heart Rhythm Disorders, South
Australian Health and Medical Research
Institute, Royal Adelaide Hospital, University of
Adelaide, Adelaide, South Australia,
Australia

BENJAMIN D. LEVINE, MD
Professor of Medicine, Institute for Exercise
and Environmental Medicine, Texas Health
Presbyterian Hospital; Department of Internal
Medicine, University of Texas Southwestern
Medical Center, Dallas, Texas

RAJIV MAHAJAN, MD, PhD
Centre for Heart Rhythm Disorders, South
Australian Health and Medical Research
Institute, Royal Adelaide Hospital, University of
Adelaide, Adelaide, South Australia, Australia

JULIE R. MCMULLEN, PhD
Baker IDI Heart and Diabetes Institute, Cardiac
Hypertrophy Laboratory; Department of
Medicine, Central Clinical School, Monash
University, Melbourne, Victoria, Australia;
Department of Physiology, Monash University,
Clayton, Victoria, Australia

ENRICA PEZZULLO, MD
Department of Cardiology, Monaldi Hospital,
Chair of Cardiology, Second University of
Naples, Naples, Italy

JURI RADMILOVIC, MD
Department of Cardiology, Monaldi Hospital,
Chair of Cardiology, Second University of
Naples, Naples, Italy

LUCIA RIEGLER, MD
Department of Cardiology, Monaldi Hospital,
Chair of Cardiology, Second University of
Naples, Naples, Italy

MARIA GIOVANNA RUSSO, MD
Professor, Department of Cardiology, Monaldi
Hospital, Second University of Naples, Naples,
Italy

SARA SABERI, MD, MS
Assistant Professor of Internal Medicine,
Division of Cardiovascular Medicine,
Department of Internal Medicine, University of
Michigan School of Medicine, Frankel
Cardiovascular Center, Ann Arbor,
Michigan

PRASHANTHAN SANDERS, MBBS, PhD
Centre for Heart Rhythm Disorders, South
Australian Health and Medical Research
Institute, Royal Adelaide Hospital, University of
Adelaide, Adelaide, South Australia,
Australia

MEGAN SANDS-LINCOLN, PhD, MPH
Elsevier Clinical Solutions, Evidence-Based
Medicine Center, Philadelphia, Pennsylvania

SATYAM SARMA, MD
Assistant Professor of Medicine, Institute for
Exercise and Environmental Medicine, Texas
Health Presbyterian Hospital; Department of
Internal Medicine, University of Texas
Southwestern Medical Center, Dallas, Texas

RAFFAELLA SCARAFILE, MD
Department of Cardiology, Monaldi Hospital,
Chair of Cardiology, Second University of
Naples, Naples, Italy

**CHRISTOPHER SEMSARIAN, MBBS, PhD,
MPH, FRACP, FAHMS, FAHA, FHRS,
FCSANZ**
Professor, Agnes Ginges Centre for Molecular
Cardiology, Centenary Institute, Newtown,
New South Wales, Australia; Sydney Medical
School, University of Sydney; Department of
Cardiology, Royal Prince Alfred Hospital,
Sydney, New South Wales, Australia

**SANJAY SHARMA, BSc, MD, FRCP (UK),
FESC**
Professor of Inherited Cardiac Diseases and
Sports Cardiology; Head of Research for the
Clinical Cardiology and Academic Group,
Cardiovascular & Cell Sciences Research
Institute, St George's University of London,
St George's University NHS Foundation Trust,
London, United Kingdom

**JOANNA SWEETING, BSc, MAppSci
(Env. Sci)**
Agnes Ginges Centre for Molecular Cardiology,
Centenary Institute, Newtown, New South
Wales, Australia; Sydney Medical School,
University of Sydney, Sydney, New South
Wales, Australia

TEE JOO YEO, MBBS, MRCP (UK)
Consultant Cardiologist, Cardiac Department,
National University Heart Centre Singapore,
Singapore, Singapore

Contents

Exercise training can have a profound effect on cardiac structure. Recent evidence suggests that the greatest determinants of exercise-induced cardiac remodeling are the intensity, duration, and frequency of training. This also has overlap with athlete fitness. There are many additional factors that are important in determining cardiac remodeling, but while further refinements evolve, the authors argue that the best means of predicting the degree of expected physiologic remodeling is to either quantify training (intensity times total training time) or its by-product (exercise capacity). A uniform approach to estimating the degree of exercise-induced cardiac remodeling will enable more consistent research.

Exercise-induced cardiac remodeling is typically an adaptive response associated with cardiac myocyte hypertrophy and renewal, increased cardiac myocyte contractility, sarcomeric remodeling, cell survival, metabolic and mitochondrial adaptations, electrical remodeling, and angiogenesis. Initiating stimuli/triggers of cardiac remodeling include increased hemodynamic load, increased sympathetic activity, and the release of hormones and growth factors. Prolonged and strenuous exercise may lead to maladaptive exercise-induced cardiac remodeling including cardiac dysfunction and arrhythmia. In addition, this article describes novel therapeutic approaches for the treatment of heart failure that target mechanisms responsible for adaptive exercise-induced cardiac remodeling, which are being developed and tested in preclinical models.

Athletes are often regarded as individuals at the pinnacle of health and fitness, nearly to the point of invincibility. The sudden cardiac death (SCD) of an athlete is therefore generally unexpected and extremely traumatic. Some of the most commonly identified causes of SCD in athletes include the genetic heart diseases. Despite thorough clinical and genetic investigation, in some cases a cause of death cannot be elucidated. Further research in these areas, spanning clinical, genetic, and public health perspectives, is required to help guide clinicians and those encountering the tragedy of SCD in an athlete.

This article summarizes the role of the 12-lead electrocardiogram (ECG) for the clinical care of athletes, with particular reference to the influence of age, gender, ethnicity, and type of sport on the appearance of the ECG, and its role in differentiating physiologic exercise-related changes from pathologic conditions implicated in sudden cardiac death (SCD). The article also explores the potential role of the ECG in detecting athletes at risk of SCD. In addition, the article reviews the evolution of ECG interpretation criteria and emphasizes the limitations of the ECG as well as the potential for future research.

Cardiac changes in athletes involve the left ventricle and atrium. Mild left atrial enlargement is common among competitive athletes, possibly a physiologic adaptation to exercise conditioning. The prevalence of this remodeling and the association with supraventricular arrhythmias has not been systematically addressed. Echocardiography screens for patients with disease involving the left atrium. New techniques like speckle tracking can recognize early atrial dysfunction and assess left atrial myocardial function in patients with either physiologic or pathologic left ventricular hypertrophy. This article reviews echocardiographic techniques in delineating the athlete's morphology and functional properties of the left atrium.

Exercise training has considerable health benefits. However, recent research has demonstrated a greater risk of atrial arrhythmias in endurance athletes. The mechanisms promoting atrial fibrillation in athletes are unclear but there seems to be a central role for atrial remodeling, accompanied by autonomic alterations and inflammation. Animal studies have provided unique insights, yet prospective human data are lacking. Treatment options seem to yield similar efficacy to that seen in a nonathletic population and may be justified as an early rhythm control strategy. Further studies are required to enhance understanding of the cardiac adaptations to intensive exercise training.

Since outcomes for patients with congenital heart disease (CHD) have greatly improved, most patients with CHD are surviving into adulthood and creating dilemmas for practitioners with regard to competitive sports participation. Much time, effort, and expertise have gone into developing the new American Heart Association/American College of Cardiology's guidelines and the European Society of Cardiology's guidelines. Practitioners should consult the guidelines but also be aware of gaps in the literature and should individualize recommendations for each patient. Both participation and restriction decisions should be made thoughtfully and collaboratively with athletes as either decision carries important consequences.

CARDIOLOGY CLINICS

ISSUE OF RELATED INTEREST

Clinics in Sports Medicine, July 2015 (Vol. 34, No. 3)
Sports Cardiology
Robert W. Battle, *Editor*
Available at: http://www.sportsmed.theclinics.com/

THE CLINICS ARE AVAILABLE ONLINE!
Access your subscription at:
www.theclinics.com

Preface
Sports Cardiology: Comprehensive Clinical Care for Athletes and Highly Active Individuals

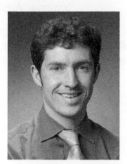
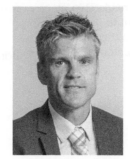

Aaron Baggish, MD, FACC, FACSM   André La Gerche, MBBS, PhD, FRACP, FESC

Editors

Competitive athletes and highly active individuals are a steadily growing segment of the global population. This growth is being driven largely by increasing recognition of the health benefits of routine vigorous physical exercise coupled with unprecedented access to competitive sporting opportunities and recreational exercise programs. Yet while lifelong commitment to physical activity is among the most powerful ways to promote health and longevity, it does not confer complete immunity and in some cases may increase the risk of cardiovascular disease. Effective clinical care of competitive athletes and highly active patients is best accomplished by combining fundamental general cardiovascular care principles with an understanding of the physiology and disease susceptibility that are unique to this population. The emerging and rapidly expanding field of sports cardiology seeks to accomplish this mission. In the clinical arena, sports cardiologists seek to integrate effective diagnostic and therapeutic strategies with

an unwavering commitment to maximizing safe and healthy athletic performance.

It is both a pleasure and an honor to introduce this issue of *Cardiology Clinics*, which is dedicated to the field of sports cardiology. In preparation for this addition of *Cardiology Clinics*, we have drawn from a rapidly growing pool of global experts in an attempt to provide timely updates on topics central to the care of the athlete. We begin with articles summarizing recent advances in the field of exercise-induced cardiac remodeling with articles focusing on molecular mechanisms, atrial adaptation, and determinants of phenotypic cardiac variability among athletes. A series of articles then addresses key clinical sports cardiology topics, including the use of the 12-lead electrocardiogram, the management of atrial fibrillation, and the application of advanced exercise testing techniques. Finally, emerging topics, including management of the athletic patient with congenital heart disease and the art and science of exercise

Cardiol Clin 34 (2016) xi–xii
http://dx.doi.org/10.1016/j.ccl.2016.08.003
0733-8651/16/© 2016 Published by Elsevier Inc.

prescription for athletic patients with cardiomyopathy, are addressed. The overarching goal of this issue of *Cardiology Clinics* is to provide the reader with a comprehensive contemporary sports cardiology resource. It is our hope that this collection of articles will further elevate the standard of care that competitive athletes and highly active patients receive worldwide. We consider ourselves privileged to have provided editorial oversight of this project and express our sincere appreciation to the contributing authors and to the readership at large for their continued commitment to the care of those who push their bodies and their minds to the limits of human performance potential.

Aaron Baggish, MD, FACC, FACSM
Cardiovascular Performance Program
Massachusetts General Hospital
Boston, MA 02114, USA

André La Gerche, MBBS, PhD, FRACP, FESC
Sports Cardiology
Baker IDI Heart and Diabetes Institute
75 Commercial Road
Melbourne 3004
Victoria, Australia

E-mail addresses:
abaggish@partners.org (A. Baggish)
Andre.lagerche@bakeridi.edu.au (A. La Gerche)

A Modern Definition of the Athlete's Heart—for Research and the Clinic

Rhys Beaudry, BSc[a,b], Mark J. Haykowsky, PhD, MSc[a,b],
Aaron Baggish, MD[c], André La Gerche, MBBS, PhD, FRACP, FESC[a,d],*

KEYWORDS

- Athlete • Heart • Cardiac • Remodeling • Hypertrophy

KEY POINTS

- There is need for a standardized framework to define the association between exercise training and the resulting changes in cardiac structure.
- There is a strong relationship between training amount (both intensity and duration), resulting fitness (often measured as Vo_{2max}) and cardiac size (volumes and mass).
- Additional factors including race, gender, and age have important influences on cardiac size.
- The relationship between training, fitness, and cardiac size can be exploited to determine whether cardiac changes are physiologically appropriate or suggestive of pathology.
- Estimates of training load and quantification of exercise conditioning are critically important factors necessary for understanding cardiac adaptation in research settings.

INTRODUCTION

Exercise can have a profound effect on cardiac size, mass, structure, and function, often referred to as the athlete's heart.[1] A consistent definition of what constitutes an athlete is essential for enabling researchers and clinicians to understand the considerable heterogeneity that exists in the literature regarding the degree of cardiac changes that may be expected as a result of exercise training. A diagnostic grey zone between athlete's heart and inherited cardiomyopathies exists at the extremes of athletic cardiac remodeling, and questions arise as to whether the observed increase in cardiac dimensions is proportional to the amount of exercise conditioning. This has

significant implications. If the cardiac remodeling is consistent with that expected for the level of training, then further investigations may not be required. Conversely, if the remodeling is greater than might be expected, then it may imply an inherited cardiomyopathy. However, it can be extremely difficult to estimate the degree of expected remodeling given the broad ranges published in the literature. For example, cardiac mass has been reported to be anywhere between 9% and 90% greater in athletes as compared with nonathletes.[2] Part of this variance may be explained by differences in measuring cardiac dimensions, but much is also likely due to differences in athletic conditioning of the cohorts encompassed under the term athlete. Current

---

Disclosures: None.
a Department of Sports Cardiology, Baker IDI Heart and Diabetes Institute, 99 Commercial Road, Melbourne 3004, Australia; b College of Nursing and Health Innovation, University of Texas at Arlington, South Nedderman Drive, Arlington, TX 76019, USA; c Division of Cardiology, Massachusetts General Hospital, 55 Fruit Street, Boston, MA 02114, USA; d Department of Cardiology, Alfred Hospital, Melbourne, Australia
* Corresponding author. Sports Cardiology, Baker IDI Heart and Diabetes Institute, Level4 Alfred Centre, 99 Commercial Road, Melbourne 3004, Australia.
E-mail address: Andre.LaGerche@bakeridi.edu.au

guidelines that attempt to define athletic status use sport-specific classifications and use exercise hemodynamics as a means of explaining the observed differences in cardiac remodeling.[3] This article discusses the strengths and weaknesses of this approach and proposes some alternate approaches for defining athletic conditioning relevant to cardiovascular adaptation.

WHAT DETERMINES CARDIAC REMODELING?

Like most biological systems, the heart adapts to the physical and metabolic load placed upon it. During dynamic exercise, the wall stress of both ventricles increases as a result of increases in pressure and volume,[4,5] and it would seem that similar hemodynamic stressors are also incurred in the atria.[6] Echocardiography and cardiac MRI have been used to demonstrate that ventricular volumes increase with exercise intensity until a point approximating anaerobic threshold, from which point ventricular volumes reduce slightly.[4,7] In a similar but not identical manner, ventricular afterload increases with exercise intensity in a near-linear manner such that the load against which the two ventricles eject increases progressively with exercise until the point of fatigue.[5,8] In combination, both a volume and pressure load are imposed on the myocardium that increases

such that the greatest load, and presumably the greatest stimulus for structural and functional adaptation, occurs during moderate-to-high intensity dynamic exercise (**Fig. 1**). A recent prospective 1-year training study supports this premise.[9]

It stands to reason that a second major determinant of the extent of cardiac remodeling would be the time that the myocardium is exposed to increased hemodynamic stress. This concept may be inferred from the finding that endurance athletes have greater cardiac remodeling when compared with athletes from sprint or team sports.[2] The observed differences in cardiac size have often been attributed to unique hemodynamic conditions created from varied combinations of static and dynamic exercise components. However, it is at least as likely that the remodeling is greater in endurance athletes simply because the hemodynamic stress is incurred for longer. For example, a typical training regime for a soccer player may involve a few hours of training per day of which the athlete may be exercising at moderate or strenuous intensity for around 60 to 90 minutes. In contrast, an endurance cyclist, rower or cross-country skier typically trains at moderate-to-high intensity for several hours each day. Thus, the cumulative time in which the heart is exposed to high hemodynamic stress is likely to be many-fold higher (**Fig. 2**). This fact, although seldom discussed in the literature, is likely to be

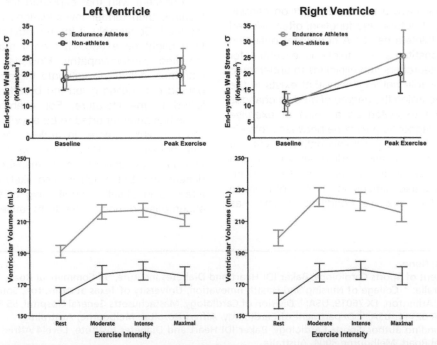

Fig. 1. A combination of invasive pressure measures and cardiac volumes obtained during exercise enable one to understand the hemodynamic stressors on the left and right ventricles. In both chambers, both the pressure and volume loads increase during exercise, and this increase is greatest at moderate to strenuous exercise intensities.

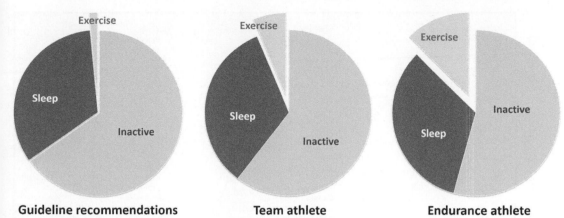

Fig. 2. Guideline recommendations (150 minutes per week of exercise) constitute approximately 2% of waking hours. Nonendurance athletes spend considerable more time exercising, but it is only the endurance athletes training more than 15 hours per week where the time spent exposed to the hemodynamic stimulus of exercise represents a significant proportion of waking hours. It seems logical that this greater proportion of exposure constitutes a greater stimulus for remodeling.

an important explanation for the greater cardiac volumes and mass observed in endurance athletes.

CRITIQUE OF THE MITCHELL CLASSIFICATION

The Mitchell criteria considers the cardiovascular impact of exercise according to the respective static and dynamic exercise components, graded from I to III and A to C, respectively (**Fig. 3**).[2] Although studies frequently categorize expected cardiac adaptation according to this schema, it is important to note that this is not the intended purpose of the Mitchell criteria. Rather, this schema was developed as a physiology guide to assist with sport eligibility and incorporates themes such as the risks associated with explosive power sports that may trigger arrhythmic events in athletes with cardiomyopathies. Although not its intended use, this schema is frequently referenced in the categorization of cardiac remodeling. However, there may be methods for simply yet accurately categorizing athletic cardiac remodeling.

The authors contend that the major determinant of cardiac remodeling is a combination of intensity, duration, and frequency of exercise training. As a result, there is also a clear overlap with fitness. Greater amounts of training at high intensity promote fitness that can be measured objectively as the maximal amount of oxygen that can be metabolized by the muscle mitochondria during exercise (Vo_{2max}). The total amount of exercise training performed at moderate or high intensity is expected to promote an increase in Vo_{2max} and cardiac remodeling. It is not surprising, therefore, that a strong correlation has been observed between cardiac size and Vo_{2max}.[10–12] Approximately 60%

to 80% of the variance in cardiac mass can be explained by fitness (**Fig. 4**), and this would suggest that fitness testing would be a reasonable means of determining whether cardiac remodeling is proportional to athletic conditioning. This can be done formally using cardiopulmonary testing to quantify Vo_{2max} or by using a number of exercise test protocols in which estimates of Vo_{2max} can be determined indirectly from treadmill or bicycle tests. From standardized tests such as the treadmill Bruce protocol, metabolic equivalents (METS) can be estimated and converted to oxygen consumption using the formula $Vo_{2max} = 3.5 \times$ METS.

Although exercise intensity, duration, and fitness can explain much of the variance in cardiac size, this is a simplified evaluation of a complex interplay between host genetic factors and environmental issues. There are many important influences on cardiac remodeling that have not been adequately considered in available data. In particular, the strong relationship between fitness and cardiac size is almost exclusively obtained from male Caucasian athletic populations. Cardiac remodeling in females is probably less profound than in males,[13] although the depth of data supporting this premise is not exhaustive. Furthermore, electrical and structural remodeling in response to an exercise stimulus appears to be more profound in black athletes, as compared with white athletes.[14–16] Furthermore, it is likely that additional genetic influences, the age of the athlete, and the cumulative years of exercise exposure influence the extent of cardiac remodeling. Thus, exercise training and resulting fitness are important determinants of athletic cardiac remodeling, but they

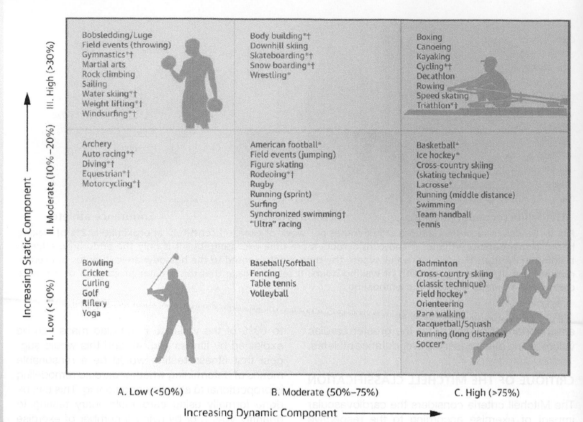

A. Low (<50%)   B. Moderate (50%–75%)   C. High (>75%)

Increasing Dynamic Component ⟶

Fig. 3. The Mitchell criteria categorize sports according to the relative amount of static and dynamic skeletal muscle usage. Although designed to provide guidance on sports participation, it has been used widely to try and explain cardiac adaptation. (*From* Levine BD, Baggish AL, Kovacs RJ, et al. Eligibility and disqualification recommendations for competitive athletes with cardiovascular abnormalities: task force 1: classification of sports: dynamic, static, and impact: a scientific statement from the American Heart Association and American College of Cardiology. J Am Coll Cardiol 2015;66(21):2350–5; with permission.)

should not be considered to the complete answer. There is ample room to further refine predictions.

In the absence of an alternative classification on which to summarize athletic cardiovascular conditioning, the utility of the Mitchell criteria has been extended to select study cohorts and to categorize athlete's heart. The underlying hypothesis justifying this practice underpinning this schema is the that of Morganroth and Maron, who drew analogies between the volume load of regurgitant valve disease

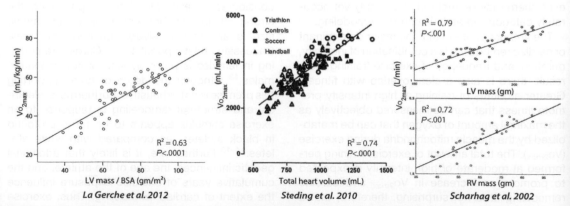

La Gerche et al. 2012   *Steding et al. 2010*   *Scharhag et al. 2002*

Fig. 4. Composite of 3 studies demonstrating a strong relationship between cardiac mass or volume and fitness measured as total oxygen consumption (Vo$_{2max}$). (*From* Refs.[10–12]; with permission.)

and that of exercise requiring concentric muscle contraction and hypothesized that endurance exercise would cause eccentric remodeling.[17,18] Conversely, they suggested that the eccentric muscle contractions required for strength and power sports induced an afterload akin to hypertension and that this would result in concentric hypertrophy. However, multiple recent studies have drawn these assumptions into question.[19–21] A prospective training study by Spence and colleagues[22] comparing endurance and strength training regimes demonstrated an increase in cardiac volumes and mass in those who performed endurance exercise but not in those who completed a strength training program. Utomi and colleagues[23] concluded similarly in a systematic review of the literature, and Luijkx and colleagues[24] observed that exercise-induced concentric remodeling was only observed in strength athletes abusing anabolic steroids and not in clean power lifters. This accumulated experience would suggest that the myocardial remodeling induced by power and strength exercise is minimal or absent. This may be due to an overestimation of the hemodynamic impact of power lifting. Although arterial blood pressures have been noted to increase substantially, this increase is only transient and is somewhat offset by the Valsalva maneuver that seems an obligatory response during maximal lifting.[25,26] There is little compelling rationale for continuing to quantify the degree of eccentric muscular activity and including this in a schema for defining the athlete's heart.

There is overlap between the Mitchell classification and a construct that defines cardiac remodeling according to the intensity and duration of exercise training. In general, those sports listed in category IIIC require significant endurance training at high intensity, and, conversely, little or no high-intensity training is required for those sports listed in category IA. However, there are a number of issues. First, all athletes performing the same sport are considered equal. In their clinical experience, the authors have observed sports persons competing in IIIC sports who are undertaking minimal training, are not particularly fit, and have little evidence of exercise-induced cardiac remodeling. At the other end of the spectrum, the have examined cricketers (a category IA sport) who undertake considerable volumes of intense training, maintain an extremely high level of fitness, and have clear evidence of athlete's heart. This individual variability would be addressed with a simple estimation of training intensity and volume or more formally with a fitness test.

The total cumulative exposure to the hemodynamic stress of high-intensity exercise is likely to be reasonably modest in some athletes classified in the highest strata of the Mitchell classification. Basketball players, ice hockey players, and boxers engage in sports in which high-intensity exercise is maintained for only minutes at a time. In contrast, training and racing in cross-country skiing involves exercise that is both high-intensity and is maintained for long periods, often a number of hours. As a result, cross-country skiers consistently rank among those with the highest fitness levels[27] and have been observed to have profound cardiac remodeling.[28,29] Thus it would seem anomalous that athletes such as cross-country skiers and basketball players, with such profoundly different training and conditioning regimes, would be categorized together in a schema designed to anticipate the degree of cardiac adaptation.

CAN WE DO BETTER?

Fig. 5 provides a simple construct for defining the association between exercise and cardiovascular adaptation. Rather than considering the type of skeletal muscle load and dichotomizing according to differences in volume and pressure load on the ventricle, this schema recognizes the fact that exercise represents both a volume and pressure load and that the magnitude of that stress is determined by exercise intensity. Thus, the expected myocardial adaptation to exercise is expected to result from the intensity of exercise and the amount of time in which that hemodynamic stress is acting on the cardiovascular system. Put simply, the stimulus for myocardial adaptation equals the hemodynamic stress (amount of intensity) times the time in which that stress is applied (duration and frequency of training).

This schema is more focused upon the individual than on the sporting discipline. Thus it recognizes the wide range of training that athletes may undertake in a given sport. Furthermore, many athletes train and compete in more than 1 sport, and this is of no significance if sport is deconstructed to its intensity and time commitment elements. Finally, a major advantage of this schema is that expected cardiac remodeling can be crudely estimated from records of exercise intensity and time or can be more accurately anticipated using measures of fitness such as a Vo_{2max} test.

RESEARCH AND THE CLINICAL IMPLICATIONS

For research applications, this is not simply a matter of semantics. An association between endurance exercise and some cardiac arrhythmias is increasingly recognized, and among the putative mechanisms underpinning this proarrhythmic tendency is

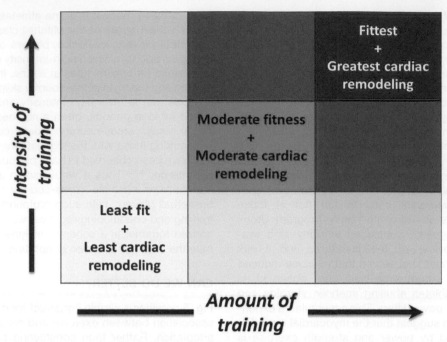

Fig. 5. The authors propose a simple schema that enables athletic cardiac remodeling to be anticipated from simple measures of exercise intensity and duration.

the degree of exercise-induced cardiac remodeling.[30] Atrial fibrillation, for example, is more prevalent among endurance athletes, and this seems to be particularly true of sports that result in the most profound ventricular and atrial remodeling. Investigators have linked atrial size to volumes of exercise and have speculated that there may be a causal relationship.[31,32] To explore this relationship with greater clarity, it would be helpful to better define the type of athlete who is most likely to have significant cardiac remodeling. We contend that this can be achieved with greater clarity using an estimate of training time and intensity. For research applications, measurements of Vo_{2max} represent an essential standard for characterizing an athletic cohort. It would be improper to study a hypertensive population without accurately quantifying blood pressure. Ideally, athletic studies should attempt to accurately define the degree of athletic conditioning.

There are also direct implications for the clinic. For example, in an athlete with an ejection fraction of 50% and an end-diastolic diameter of 65 mm, it is necessary to differentiate between athlete's heart and an early dilated cardiomyopathy.[1] There are a number of modern imaging techniques that may aid in this assessment,[33] but a logical first assessment would be to perform an exercise test and see whether the athlete's fitness (eg, Vo_{2max}) is commensurate with the cardiac enlargement. As detailed in **Fig. 4**, there are already reasonably strong data from multiple investigators from which

to define the relationship between Vo_{2max} and cardiac volumes or mass.[10–12] Secondly, the suggested exercise schema can be used to advise patients who have a cardiac pathology for which exercise restriction is prudent. Patients can find it difficult to understand guidance based on the Mitchell criteria. For example, the patient with hypertrophic cardiomyopathy may be advised that he or she can only compete in class IA sports that imply that any significant physical exertion incurs risk. The patient then asks whether he or she can ride his or her bike to work and at what intensity. A simple recommendation explaining the interaction between exercise duration and intensity can be a useful way of providing an exercise prescription that is logical and measurable and can be applied across sporting disciplines.

SUMMARY

The modern definition of the athlete's heart should no longer be defined by outdated concepts of volume and pressure load. The effect of strength and power training on cardiovascular adaptation has repeatedly been demonstrated to be many fold less important than exercise intensity and exercise duration. Thus, the authors propose that investigators and clinicians consider a much simpler appreciation of the athlete's heart, defined by the 2 simple variables of exercise intensity and duration. The result can be measured by testing fitness and seems to be more closely associated with cardio-vascular remodeling than does categorization according to sporting discipline. There are limitations of this concept; notably the influences of ethnicity, age, and gender are yet to be incorporated. However, this new schema can be incorporated into research applications and provides a simple framework to assist with clinical decision making.

REFERENCES

1. Prior DL, La Gerche A. The athlete's heart. Heart 2012;98(12):947–55.
2. Pluim BM, Zwinderman AH, van der Laarse A, et al. The athlete's heart. A meta-analysis of cardiac structure and function. Circulation 2000;101(3):336–44.
3. Levine BD, Baggish AL, Kovacs RJ, et al. Eligibility and disqualification recommendations for competitive athletes with cardiovascular abnormalities: task force 1: classification of sports: dynamic, static, and impact: a scientific statement from the American Heart Association and American College of Cardiology. Circulation 2015;132(22):e262–6.
4. La Gerche A, Claessen G, Dymarkowski S, et al. Exercise-induced right ventricular dysfunction is associated with ventricular arrhythmias in endurance athletes. Eur Heart J 2015;36(30):1998–2010.
5. La Gerche A, Heidbuchel H, Burns AT, et al. Disproportionate exercise load and remodeling of the athlete's right ventricle. Med Sci Sports Exerc 2011; 43(6):974–81.
6. Gabrielli L, Bijnens BH, Brambila C, et al. Differential atrial performance at rest and exercise in athletes: potential trigger for developing atrial dysfunction? Scand J Med Sci Sports 2016. [Epub ahead of print].
7. Haykowsky MJ, Brubaker PH, John JM, et al. Determinants of exercise intolerance in elderly heart failure patients with preserved ejection fraction. J Am Coll Cardiol 2011;58(3):265–74.
8. Claessen G, La Gerche A, Voigt JU, et al. Accuracy of echocardiography to evaluate pulmonary vascular and RV function during exercise. JACC Cardiovasc Imaging 2016;9(5):532–43.
9. Arbab-Zadeh A, Perhonen M, Howden E, et al. Cardiac remodeling in response to 1 year of intensive endurance training. Circulation 2014;130(24):2152–61.
10. Steding K, Engblom H, Buhre T, et al. Relation between cardiac dimensions and peak oxygen uptake. J Cardiovasc Magn Reson 2010;12(1):8.
11. La Gerche A, Burns AT, Taylor AJ, et al. Maximal oxygen consumption is best predicted by measures of cardiac size rather than function in healthy adults. Eur J Appl Physiol 2012;112(6):2139–47.
12. Scharhag J, Schneider G, Urhausen A, et al. Athlete's heart: right and left ventricular mass and function in male endurance athletes and untrained

13. Howden EJ, Perhonen M, Peshock RM, et al. Females have a blunted cardiovascular response to one year of intensive supervised endurance training. J Appl Physiol (1985) 2015;119(1):37–46.
14. Basavarajaiah S, Boraita A, Whyte G, et al. Ethnic differences in left ventricular remodeling in highly-trained athletes relevance to differentiating physiologic left ventricular hypertrophy from hypertrophic cardiomyopathy. J Am Coll Cardiol 2008;51(23):2256–62.
15. Papadakis M, Carre F, Kervio G, et al. The prevalence, distribution, and clinical outcomes of electrocardiographic repolarization patterns in male athletes of African/Afro-Caribbean origin. Eur Heart J 2011;32(18):2304–13.
16. Rawlins J, Carre F, Kervio G, et al. Ethnic differences in physiological cardiac adaptation to intense physical exercise in highly trained female athletes. Circulation 2010;121(9):1078–85.
17. Morganroth J, Maron BJ, Henry WL, et al. Comparative left ventricular dimensions in trained athletes. Ann Intern Med 1975;82(4):521–4.
18. Morganroth J, Maron BJ. The athlete's heart syndrome: a new perspective. Ann N Y Acad Sci 1977;301:931–41.
19. Haykowsky MJ, Tomczak CR. LV hypertrophy in resistance or endurance trained athletes: the Morganroth hypothesis is obsolete, most of the time. Heart 2014;100(16):1225–6.
20. Haykowsky MJ, Quinney HA, Gillis R, et al. Left ventricular morphology in junior and master resistance trained athletes. Med Sci Sports Exerc 2000;32(2): 349–52.
21. Haykowsky MJ, Gillis R, Quinney A, et al. Left ventricular morphology in elite female resistance-trained athletes. Am J Cardiol 1998;82(7):912–4.
22. Spence AL, Carter HH, Naylor LH, et al. A prospective randomized longitudinal study involving 6 months of endurance or resistance exercise. Conduit artery adaptation in humans. J Physiol 2013;591(Pt 5): 1265–75.
23. Utomi V, Oxborough D, Whyte GP, et al. Systematic review and meta-analysis of training mode, imaging modality and body size influences on the morphology and function of the male athlete's heart. Heart 2013; 99(23):1727–33.
24. Luijkx T, Velthuis BK, Backx FJ, et al. Anabolic androgenic steroid use is associated with ventricular dysfunction on cardiac MRI in strength trained athletes. Int J Cardiol 2013;167(3):664–8.
25. MacDougall JD, McKelvie RS, Moroz DE, et al. Factors affecting blood pressure during heavy weight lifting and static contractions. J Appl Physiol (1985) 1992;73(4):1590–7.
26. Haykowsky M, Taylor D, Teo K, et al. Left ventricular wall stress during leg-press exercise performed

with a brief Valsalva maneuver. Chest 2001;119(1): 150–4.

27. Spencer MD, Murias JM, Grey TM, et al. Regulation of VO(2) kinetics by O(2) delivery: insights from acute hypoxia and heavy-intensity priming exercise in young men. J Appl Physiol (1985) 2012;112(6): 1023–32.

28. Grimsmo J, Grundvold I, Maehlum S, et al. High prevalence of atrial fibrillation in long-term endurance cross-country skiers: echocardiographic findings and possible predictors—a 28-30 years follow-up study. Eur J Cardiovasc Prev Rehabil 2010;17(1): 100–5.

29. Henriksen E, Landelius J, Wesslen L, et al. Echocardiographic right and left ventricular measurements in male elite endurance athletes. Eur Heart J 1996; 17(7):1121–8.

30. La Gerche A, Heidbuchel H. Can intensive exercise harm the heart? You can get too much of a good thing. Circulation 2014;130(12):992–1002.

31. Grimsmo J, Grundvold I, Maehlum S, et al. Echocardiographic evaluation of aged male cross country skiers. Scand J Med Sci Sports 2011;21(3):412–9.

32. Wilhelm M, Roten L, Tanner H, et al. Atrial remodeling, autonomic tone, and lifetime training hours in nonelite athletes. Am J Cardiol 2011;108(4):580–5.

33. La Gerche A, Baggish AL, Knuuti J, et al. Cardiac imaging and stress testing asymptomatic athletes to identify those at risk of sudden cardiac death. JACC Cardiovasc Imaging 2013;6(9):993–1007.

Molecular Aspects of Exercise-induced Cardiac Remodeling

Bianca C. Bernardo, PhD[a], Julie R. McMullen, PhD[a,b,c],*

KEYWORDS

- Exercise • Cardiac remodeling • Molecular mechanisms • Cardiac myocyte • Cardiac hypertrophy
- Drug targets

KEY POINTS

- Cardiac enlargement that occurs in response to moderate exercise is typically considered an adaptive physiologic response that is associated with normal or improved cardiac function. This adaptive remodeling is associated with cardiac myocyte hypertrophy and renewal (proliferation and increased endogenous cardiac stem cells), increased cardiac myocyte contractility, sarcomeric remodeling, cell survival, metabolic and mitochondrial adaptations, electrical remodeling, and angiogenesis.
- At the molecular level, adaptive exercise-induced cardiac remodeling has been associated with signaling pathways/modulators activated by growth factors, hormones (growth and thyroid), and mechanical stretch, including the insulin-like growth factor 1 receptor–phosphoinositide 3-kinase–phosphoinositide-dependent protein kinase-1–protein kinase B signaling pathway, β-adrenoreceptors, transcription factors (eg, CCAAT/enhancer-binding protein β, heat shock factor 1), and microRNAs (eg, miR-222).
- By contrast, intense endurance exercise has been associated with some adverse cardiac remodeling, cardiac dysfunction, and arrhythmia. This cardiac remodeling may be more similar at the cellular and molecular levels to disease-induced pathologic remodeling. Molecular mechanisms implicated include β_1-adrenoreceptor desensitization, and prolonged tumor necrosis factor α-nuclear factor kappa B–p38 signaling.
- Novel therapeutic approaches for the treatment of heart failure that target mechanisms responsible for adaptive exercise-induced cardiac remodeling are being developed and tested in preclinical models.

INTRODUCTION

Cardiac remodeling is the result of molecular and cellular changes that manifest clinically as changes in the size, shape, and function of the heart. In response to exercise training, all 4 chambers of the heart can enlarge (left and right atria, and left ventricle [LV], and right ventricle [RV]).[1–3] However, to date, cellular and molecular mechanisms have mainly been studied in the LV. Initiating stimuli/triggers of exercise-induced remodeling include increased hemodynamic load, increased sympathetic activity, and the release of hormones and growth factors, all of which activate multiple molecular pathways. The activation of signaling cascades affects

Disclosure: The authors have nothing to disclose.
[a] Baker IDI Heart and Diabetes Institute, Cardiac Hypertrophy Laboratory, PO Box 6492, Melbourne, VIC 3004, Australia; [b] Department of Medicine, Central Clinical School, Monash University, 99 Commercial Road, Melbourne, VIC 3004, Australia; [c] Department of Physiology, Monash University, Wellington Road, Clayton, VIC 3800, Australia
* Corresponding author. Baker IDI Heart and Diabetes Institute, Cardiac Hypertrophy Laboratory, PO Box 6492, Melbourne, Victoria 3004, Australia.
E-mail address: julie.mcmullen@bakeridi.edu.au

Cardiol Clin 34 (2016) 515–530
http://dx.doi.org/10.1016/j.ccl.2016.06.002
0733-8651/16/© 2016 Elsevier Inc. All rights reserved.

multiple processes within different cardiac cell types (eg, cardiac myocytes, fibroblasts, endothelial cells, vascular smooth muscle cells). Cardiac remodeling in response to exercise is generally considered an adaptive response and distinct from the remodeling that occurs in heart disease settings.[4,5] However, it is also recognized that prolonged strenuous exercise can lead to adverse cardiac remodeling and complications such as arrhythmia.[6] To date, the cellular and molecular mechanisms responsible for adaptive heart growth (ie, physiologic hypertrophy) in response to moderate exercise training are better characterized and are the focus of this article (**Table 1**). However, this article also describes what is currently known in relation to the molecular mechanisms that contribute to adverse remodeling in response to prolonged high-intensity exercise (see **Table 1**). In addition, this article discusses novel therapeutic approaches for the treatment of heart failure that target mechanisms responsible for adaptive exercise-induced cardiac remodeling.

MOLECULAR MECHANISMS ASSOCIATED WITH ADAPTIVE EXERCISE-INDUCED CARDIAC REMODELING

Exercise represents a dynamic and intermittent stimulus associated with increased sympathetic activity (release of catecholamines: norepinephrine/noradrenaline, epinephrine/adrenaline), mechanical stress, altered release of hormones (eg, growth hormone [GH] and thyroid hormone [TH]), and the increased production and secretion of several growth factors. Growth factors that have been associated with exercise training or fitness include insulin-like growth factor 1 (IGF1), hepatocyte growth factor (HGF), platelet-derived growth factor (PDGF), vascular endothelial growth factor (VEGF), and neuregulin-1 (NRG1).[2,7,8] These stimuli subsequently activate numerous signaling cascades within the heart, leading to processes such as cardiac myocyte hypertrophy and renewal/proliferation, cardiac myocyte contractility, sarcomeric remodeling, extracellular matrix (ECM) remodeling, cell survival, angiogenesis, electrical

Table 1
Cellular and molecular features associated with adaptive and maladaptive exercise-induced remodeling

Cellular and Molecular Mechanisms Associated with Adaptive Exercise-induced Remodeling	Cellular and Molecular Mechanisms Associated with Maladaptive Exercise-induced Remodeling
Cellular	Cellular
• Cardiac myocyte hypertrophy and renewal	• Cardiac myocyte hypertrophy
• ↑ eCSCs (proliferation and differentiation)	• No or ↑ fibrosis
• ↑ myocyte contractility and sarcomere remodeling	• ↑ inflammation
• ↑ angiogenesis	
• No fibrosis	
• No or ↓ apoptosis	
• ↑ mitochondrial biogenesis	
Stimuli and molecular mechanisms	Stimuli and molecular mechanisms
• Intermittent release of hormones (eg, GH, TH) and growth factors (eg, IGF1, VEGF, NRG1, HGF)	• More prolonged release of factors; eg, TNFα
• Intermittent ↑ catecholamines and activation of β-ARs	• More prolonged ↑ catecholamines and eventual desensitization of β-ARs
• IGF1R-PI3K-PDK1-Akt (other regulators of pathway: PAK1, PRAS40)	• ↑ oxidative stress
• VEGF-PI3K-Akt-eNOS	• Activation of NFκB-p38 MAPK
• Akt-C/EBPβ-CITED4	• Possible release of ET-1 and TGFβ from cardiac cells (eg, myocytes, immune and vascular) and activation of GPCR signaling cascades
• HSF1	
• miR-222	

Abbreviations: β-AR, β-adrenergic receptor; Akt1, protein kinase B; C/EBPβ, CCAAT/enhancer-binding protein β; CITED4, CBP/p300-interacting transactivator 4; eCSCs, endogenous cardiac stem/progenitor cells; eNOS, endothelial nitric oxide synthase; ET-1, endothelin-1; GH, growth hormone; GPCR, G protein–coupled receptor; HGF, hepatocyte growth factor; HSF1, heat shock factor 1; IGF1, insulin-like growth factor 1; IGF1R, insulin-like growth factor 1 receptor; MAPK, mitogen activated protein kinase; miR, microRNA; NFκB, nuclear factor kappa-light-chain-enhancer of activated B cells; NRG1, neuregulin-1; PAK1, p21 protein (Cdc42/Rac)-activated kinase 1; PDK1, phosphoinositide-dependent protein kinase-1; PI3K, phosphoinositide 3-kinase; PRAS40, proline rich Akt substrate; TGFβ, transforming growth factor beta; TH, thyroid hormone; TNFα, tumor necrosis factor α; VEGF, vascular endothelial growth factor.

remodeling, and metabolic/mitochondrial adaptations (**Fig. 1**). The role of individual factors and genes regulating these processes has been assessed using animal models. The most common exercise models used to examine molecular mechanisms responsible for adaptive heart growth include rodents subjected to swim training, and voluntary free wheel and treadmill running (**Table 2**).

Adaptive exercise-induced cardiac remodeling is associated with numerous mechanisms. This article focuses on those studies in which molecular mechanisms have been identified and shown to have a causal role using genetic models/tools (summary provided in **Table 1** and signaling cascades presented in **Fig. 2**).

Cardiac Myocyte Hypertrophy and Renewal/Proliferation

Hypertrophy of cardiac myocytes has been considered the dominant contributor to cardiac enlargement because most adult myocytes are unable to proliferate or be renewed.[9–11] Consequently, in most of the studies described in the subsequent text of this article, cardiac myocyte proliferation or renewal were not specifically examined. However, it is now recognized that exercise may lead to cardiac myocyte proliferation and renewal in a small percentage of cells,[12–14] and studies examining both hypertrophy and myocyte proliferation are also highlighted later.

The role of the IGF1–phosphoinositide 3-kinase (PI3K)-phosphoinositide–dependent protein kinase-1 (PDK1)–protein kinase B (Akt1) pathway in contributing to cardiac myocyte hypertrophy has received particular attention because this pathway is recognized to control cell and organ size.[15] Furthermore, the cardiac formation of IGF1 was shown to be higher in elite soccer players with physiologic hypertrophy; other factors associated with disease-induced pathologic hypertrophy, such as angiotensin II and endothelin-1, remained unchanged.[16] Genetic mouse models (cardiac-specific/global) have been used to assess the role of the insulin-like growth factor 1 receptor (IGF1R)–PI3K-PDK1-Akt1 pathway mediating exercise-induced cardiac hypertrophy (see **Fig. 2**). Mice with deletion or reduced activity of IGF1R, PI3K, PDK1, and Akt1 all displayed a blunted hypertrophic response to swim exercise training.[17–22] Several PI3K classes and isoforms exist.[4] PI3K(p110α) seems to be the dominant

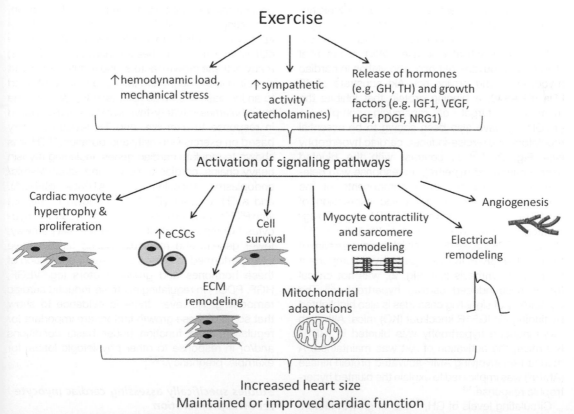

Fig. 1. An overview of exercise-induced stimuli/triggers and the cellular responses that accompany adaptive exercise-induced cardiac remodeling. eCSCs, endogenous cardiac stem/progenitor cells.

Table 2
Characteristics of animal models used to study adaptive and maladaptive exercise-induced remodeling

Animal Models Used to Study Adaptive Exercise-induced Remodeling	Animal Models to Study Maladaptive Exercise-induced Remodeling

• Swim exercise training for 2–5 wk (90-min sessions twice a day, 5–7 d/wk). Typically, a ramp protocol starting at 10 min twice a day
   Phenotype
      ↑ heart mass
      Normal/↑ function
	• Swim training or treadmill running for 6 wk. VO_2 max >70%
	   Phenotype
	      No change in heart mass
	      No change in function
	      ↑ atrial weight
	      Atrial fibrosis
	      Atrial inflammation
	      ↑ susceptibility to AF

• Voluntary free wheel running for 4–8 wk
   Phenotype
      ↑ heart mass
      Normal/↑↑function	

• Treadmill running for 4–6 wk (60 min/d, 5–7 d/wk). Typically, a ramp protocol starting at 10 min/d and <70% VO_2 max
   Phenotype
      ↑ heart mass
      Normal/↑ function
	• Treadmill running for 16 wk (60 min/d, 5 d/wk).
	   Phenotype
	      ↑ heart mass
	      ↓ systolic function
	      ↓ diastolic function
	      RV fibrosis

Abbreviations: AF, atrial fibrillation; VO_2 max, maximal oxygen uptake.
Data from Refs.[14,17,20,22,24,27,47,95,98]

isoform regulating exercise-induced physiologic hypertrophy, but PI3K(p110β) has also been implicated.[17,20] Other regulators of this pathway, including P21-activated kinase (PAK1; a potential PDK2 that regulates Akt phosphorylation in cardiac myocytes[23]) and proline rich Akt substrate of 40 kDa (PRAS40; a binding protein that inhibits the mammalian target of rapamycin complex 1 [mTORC1]) have also been shown to be essential regulators of exercise-induced cardiac hypertrophy (see **Fig. 2**).[24,25] In contrast with the blunted exercise-induced hypertrophic response with deletion/reduced expression of components of the IGF1 pathway, increased cardiac expression of IGF1R or Akt (via deletion of PHLPP1) led to an exaggerated hypertrophic response to swim training.[26,27] Ribosomal S6 kinase (S6K), which is downstream of the IGF1R-PI3K-PDK1-Akt1 pathway and important for protein synthesis (see **Fig. 2**), was not critical for exercise-induced cardiac hypertrophy.[28] The complexity of signaling cascades is also highlighted by findings in IGF1R knockout (KO) mice. Although swim-induced hypertrophy was blunted in IGF1R KO mice, the activation of Akt was maintained. A mechanism involving AMP-activated protein kinase (AMPK) was implicated to explain the blunted hypertrophic response.[19]

Circulating levels of GH,[29] and of growth factors including PDGF, transforming growth factor-β (TGFβ), VEGF, and HGF, have also been shown to be increased in response to exercise.[7,8] In addition, circulating levels of NRG1β (a member of the epidermal growth factor family) were positively associated with fitness in healthy humans.[30] Of note, many of these growth factors also regulate PI3K/Akt signaling in the heart, and increased GH levels lead to an increase in cardiac IGF1 (see **Fig. 2**).[31–34] The hypothalamus-pituitary-thyroid axis is also activated in response to exercise, and TH levels can vary based on exercise intensity and duration.[35] TH was shown to regulate cardiac genes, including myosin heavy chains, cardiac troponin, and sarcoplasmic/endoplasmic reticulum Ca^{2+}-ATPase (SERCA), and a TH receptor (TRα1) was shown to interact with PI3K to induce protein synthesis in cardiac myocytes.[4] Compared with the IGF1-PI3K-Akt pathway, fewer genetic and molecular-based studies have been performed to assess the direct contribution of these hormones and growth factors (eg, VEGF, HGF, PDGF) in regulating exercise-induced cardiac remodeling. However, there is evidence to show that some of these growth factors are important for regulating heart function under basal conditions and/or in response to other physiologic loads; for example, pregnancy.[30,36]

Studies specifically assessing cardiac myocyte renewal/proliferation

In some disease settings and in response to exercise, the heart seems to have the capacity to produce new cardiac myocytes either from endogenous cardiac stem/progenitor cells (eCSCs) or preexisting cardiac myocytes.[2,37–39] Exercise-induced hypertrophy (treadmill running or swim training) was shown to be associated with increased numbers of eCSCs,[12,13,39] and in some cases the differentiation of eCSCs into cardiac myocytes and capillaries was implicated (see **Fig. 2**).[13] Waring and colleagues[13] described the identification of new cardiac myocytes in a dose-dependent manner in rats subjected to low-intensity and high-intensity treadmill running for 4 weeks (high-intensity exercise in this study was not representative of strenuous endurance training associated with adverse outcomes; the model was associated with enhanced systolic function). The high-intensity model was associated with cardiac enlargement caused by cardiac myocyte hypertrophy and new cardiac myocyte formation (approximately 7%), which was attributed to proliferation and differentiation of eCSCs.[13] Increased sympathetic activity (activating β_2-adrenoreceptors [AR] on eCSCs) and IGF1, NRG1, and HGF have been implicated for inducing eCSC proliferation,[13,39] whereas bone morphogenetic protein 10 and TGF-β1 have been shown to stimulate the differentiation of eCSCs into cardiac lineages (see **Fig. 2**).[2,13] However, because apoptosis and/or necrosis rates are unchanged or reduced in settings of physiologic hypertrophy,[40–42] and eCSCs may be in a protected microenvironment because of the presence of growth factors released with exercise, it is possible that the increased numbers of eCSCs are also a consequence of reduced apoptosis/necrosis.[12] These mechanisms have not been assessed in detail in these studies. Fate mapping studies will be required to definitively identify the source of new cardiac myocytes in response to exercise.[43]

In another study, swim training–induced hypertrophy was associated with cardiac myocyte hypertrophy and proliferation. Mechanistically, this was caused, at least in part, by reduced expression of the transcription factor CCAAT/enhancer-binding protein β (C/EBPβ) and increased CBP/p300-interacting transactivator 4 (CITED4).[14] Akt was shown to be an upstream regulator of C/EBPβ.[14] Note that it has also been suggested that GH (which increased cardiac IGF1 levels) can stimulate cardiac myocyte proliferation in the adult rat heart,[32] and cardiac transgenic expression of PI3K was shown to regulate C/EBPβ and CITED4 expression.[44] Heterozygote C/EBPβ mice with reduced cardiac C/EBPβ showed heart enlargement associated with cardiac myocyte hypertrophy and proliferation, and improved fractional shortening (ie, a phenotype resembling that observed in exercise-trained wild-type mice). Heterozygote C/EBPβ mice showed an increase in exercise capacity under basal conditions, but the hypertrophic response to swim training was not augmented.[14] Serum response factor and Gata4 were implicated downstream of C/EBPβ in mediating hypertrophy. Transcription factors such as GATA4 have been shown to participate in both adaptive and maladaptive cardiac hypertrophy,[45] although the effect of GATA4 deletion on swim-induced cardiac hypertrophy seems modest compared with a reduction of PI3K or Akt.[17,18,45] Furthermore, although GATA4 is activated in a setting of IGF1R-induced hypertrophy, it is not required for the hypertrophic response,[46] suggesting that other transcription factors are involved. Levels of another transcription factor, heat shock factor 1 (HSF1), were increased in the heart in response to voluntary wheel running. Using HSF1-deficient heterozygote mice, it was shown that HSF1 is important for maintaining cardiac function in a setting of exercise but had no effect on the hypertrophic growth.[47]

Cardiac Myocyte Contractility and Sarcomeric Remodeling

In response to exercise, heart rate and cardiac contractility increase to meet the metabolic demands of the body. This increase is facilitated by increased cardiac myocyte contraction, which is achieved, in part, by the increased release of stored calcium (Ca^{2+}) within the sarcoplasmic reticulum (SR) binding to components of the contractile apparatus and sarcomeric remodeling.[48,49]

An array of genetic mouse models, and studies on isolated cardiac myocytes from exercise-trained rodents suggest that cardiac contractility is increased via the following mechanisms: increased Ca^{2+} entry into cardiac myocytes via L-type Ca^{2+} channels (LTCC), stimulation of β_1-AR (caused by exercise-induced catecholamine release), generation of cyclic AMP, activation of protein kinase A (PKA), increased SR Ca^{2+} (involving SERCA and the phosphorylation status of phospholamban [PLN]; regulated by Ca^{2+}/calmodulin-dependent kinase II [CaMKII]), and increased Ca^{2+} release via the ryanodine receptor/calcium release channel (RyR2).[48,50,51] Ca^{2+} released into the cytosol then enables sarcomere shortening and contraction.

In response to an increased load with exercise, cardiac myocytes also synthesize new contractile proteins and assemble new sarcomeres. The lateral borders of sarcomeres are delineated by Z discs. Z discs were initially considered to largely provide structural integrity. However, it is now

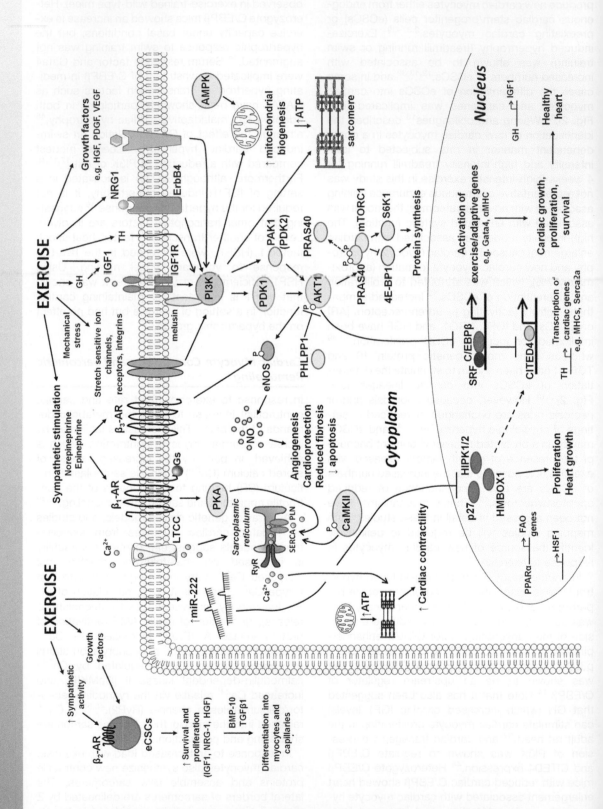

recognized that the Z disc represents a nodal hub of signaling, converting mechanical signals into chemical signals, and leading to transcriptional responses. Exercise is known to regulate components of the contractile apparatus.[48] However, molecular-based studies delineating specific mechanisms are currently limited. Using cardiac-specific transgenic mouse models with increased or decreased PI3K activity, Waardenberg and colleagues[52] showed that PI3K regulates key components of the Z disc and costamere, including melusin (see **Fig. 2**).[52]

Extracellular Matrix Remodeling

In cardiac disease settings, cardiac myocyte growth is typically accompanied by cardiac fibrosis (ie, excessive synthesis of ECM; eg, collagens by cardiac fibroblasts), and this leads to cardiac stiffening. By contrast, the regulation of the ECM in response to exercise training typically occurs in a coordinated fashion, allowing a structural framework for the coordination of mechanical, electrical, and chemical processes to maintain normal cardiac contractility. Compared with the molecular mechanisms responsible for cardiac myocyte biology, less is known regarding the exact mechanisms that regulate fibroblast biology in settings of health and disease.[53] However, there is evidence to suggest that factors released from cardiac myocytes play a role in regulating the ECM response. For instance, IGF1-PI3K signaling within cardiac myocytes was important for normal ECM deposition and protection against cardiac fibrosis in cardiac disease settings.[17,54,55]

Cell Survival

Unlike the diseased heart, which is associated with increased apoptosis,[4] exercise training has been accompanied by unchanged or decreased levels/rates of apoptotic markers.[40–42] Exercise is known to have antiapoptotic effects via activation of Akt and endothelial nitric oxide synthase (eNOS) (see **Fig. 2**).[4,42]

Metabolic and Mitochondrial Adaptations

Mitochondria play an essential role in energy production. The heart derives most of its energy from fatty acids (FAs), with glucose and lactate providing the remaining sources.[56] To preserve or enhance cardiac metabolism, exercise training has been accompanied by increased fatty acid and glucose oxidation, increased mitochondrial biogenesis, induction of FA oxidation pathways regulated by AMPK and peroxisome proliferator activated receptor-α (PPARα), and increased expression of lipogenic genes.[4,22,57] PI3K was shown to be essential for exercise-induced mitochondrial adaptations, but this was independent of Akt and PDK1.[21,22]

The effects of exercise on the generation of reactive oxygen species from mitochondria and alterations to the antioxidant capacity of the heart have been inconsistent. However, there seems to be growing support for the idea that exercise-induced changes to antioxidant enzymes contribute to adaptive exercise-induced remodeling and an increase in the antioxidative defense system.[58–60]

Electrical Remodeling

In a setting of exercise-induced hypertrophy it is crucial that the density of ion channels on cardiac myocytes increases in proportion to cardiac myocyte hypertrophy to maintain myocardial excitability. In a mouse model of swim-induced hypertrophy, electrical function was preserved, and this was accompanied by increased K^+ currents, increased depolarizing Ca^{2+} currents, and an upregulation of the expression of corresponding cardiac ion channels.[61] A similar observation

---

Fig. 2. Signaling pathways implicated in mediating exercise-induced cardiac remodeling. Signaling within cardiac myocytes are mainly highlighted but some pathways are relevant to other cardiac cells types (eg, Akt-eNOS-NO in vascular cells). 4E-BP1, eukaryotic translation initiation factor 4E–binding protein 1; αMHC, α-myosin heavy chain; β-AR, β-adrenergic receptor; Akt1, protein kinase B; AMPK, AMP-activated protein kinase; BMP-10, bone morphogenetic protein 10; CaMKII, calcium/calmodulin-dependent protein kinase II; C/EBPβ, CCAAT/enhancer-binding protein β; CITED4, CBP/p300-interacting transactivator 4; eNOS, endothelial nitric oxide synthase; ErbB4, erb-b2 receptor tyrosine kinase 4; FAO, fatty acid oxidation; GATA, GATA binding protein; HIPK1/2, homeodomain interacting protein kinase 1/2; HMBOX1, homeobox-containing protein 1; HSF1, heat shock factor 1; IGF1R, insulin-like growth factor 1 receptor; LTCC, L-type calcium channel; mTORC1, mammalian target of rapamycin complex 1; NO, nitric oxide; P, phosphorylation; PAK1, p21 protein (Cdc42/Rac)–activated kinase 1; PDK1/2, phosphoinositide-dependent protein kinase-1/2; PHLPP1, PH domain and leucine-rich repeat protein phosphatase 1; PI3K, phosphoinositide 3-kinase; PKA, protein kinase A; PLN, phospholamban; PPARα, peroxisome proliferator activated receptor alpha; PRAS40, proline rich AKT substrate; RyR, ryanodine receptor; S6K1, ribosomal protein s6 kinase 1; SERCA, sarcoplasmic/endoplasmic reticulum Ca^{2+}-ATPase; SRF, serum response factor; TGFβ1, transforming growth factor beta 1.

was reported in transgenic mice with physiologic hypertrophy caused by increased expression of PI3K.[61] Thus, electrical remodeling in response to exercise may be mediated in part by PI3K.

Angiogenesis and Vascular Remodeling

In response to exercise, blood vessels proliferate by sprouting from existing vessels (ie, angiogenesis) and can undergo changes in phenotype (ie, vascular remodeling). Increased angiogenesis is considered an integral response for maintaining perfusion and an adequate nutrient supply for processes such as cardiac myocyte hypertrophy.[62,63] VEGF is secreted in response to exercise, is a potent factor for promoting angiogenesis, and can activate PI3K-Akt signaling (see **Fig. 2**).[2,64] Muscle-specific VEGF deficiency (heart and skeletal muscle) led to reduced capillary density in skeletal and cardiac muscle, cardiac dysfunction, and exercise intolerance.[65] However, this study was confounded by the deletion of VEGF from skeletal muscle in addition to cardiac muscle. Note that transgenic-induced activation of PI3K within cardiac myocytes but not Akt was sufficient for maintaining or enhancing myocardial capillary density in a setting of physiologic cardiac hypertrophy.[44,66] In the Akt model, transgenic expression for 2 weeks led to physiologic hypertrophy associated with preserved contractile function. However, by 6 weeks, transgenic expression of Akt was associated with depressed systolic function and reduced capillary density.[66]

eNOS activation and nitric oxide (NO) generation are also considered to play an important role in mediating the cardioprotective vascular effects of exercise. Exercise is hypothesized to increase eNOS and NO production via at least 2 mechanisms. First, exercise leads to an increase in vascular wall stress. Fluid shear stress was shown to activate PI3K-Akt signaling, increase activity of vascular eNOS and NO production, and protect against apoptosis (see **Fig. 2**).[67,68] Second, exercise training also leads to an increase in the circulating levels of catecholamines, which activates ARs and downstream signaling. Mice subjected to voluntary free wheel running for 4 weeks had increased circulating levels of epinephrine and norepinephrine, increased abundance of β_3-ARs, activation of cardiac eNOS and NO generation, and were protected against ischemia-reperfusion injury (see **Fig. 2**). Using β_3-AR–deficient mice it was shown that the eNOS-NO generation and protection were mediated in part by β_3-AR stimulation.[69]

Emerging Role of microRNAs in Exercise-induced Cardiac Remodeling

MicroRNAs (miRNAs) are non–protein coding small RNAs that regulate gene expression networks and play important roles in cardiovascular biology and disease.[70,71] Several studies have investigated the impact of exercise on miRNA expression in the heart or within the circulation. In response to swim or run training in rodents, or a transgenic mouse model with physiologic hypertrophy (caused by increased PI3K activity), some distinct miRNA signatures were identified and may contribute to the cardiovascular adaptive response to exercise by regulating target genes associated with cardiac biology (differentially regulated miRNAs and targets have been listed in several articles/reviews).[72–78] For example, miR-29c expression increased in response to aerobic exercise training and correlated with a decrease in 2 targets: collagen I and III.[79] Other studies have shown that acute and chronic bouts of exercise impart differential changes in miRNA expression (reviewed in detail elsewhere[73,80,81]). However, understanding of the functional roles of these miRNAs is only just emerging. To date, miR-222 is the only miRNA shown to be necessary for exercise-induced heart growth.[75] miR-222 was upregulated in the hearts of exercised mice subjected to swimming or voluntary wheel running, as well as in the circulation of patients with heart failure after exercise testing on a bicycle ergometer. Further, inhibition of miR-222 (using miRNA inhibitors) in mice prevented an increase in heart size induced by swim training, showing that miR-222 was necessary for exercise-induced heart growth.[75] Mechanistically, cardiac myocyte proliferation and regulation of miR-222 target genes (p27, a cell-cycle inhibitor, and homeobox-containing protein 1, a transcriptional repressor) and CITED4 were implicated (see **Fig. 2**).[75] Note that transgenic cardiac-overexpression of miR-222 in mice was not sufficient to recapitulate the exercised-heart phenotype under basal conditions. However, 6 weeks after ischemic injury, transgenic miR-222 mice were protected against pathologic cardiac remodeling. Thus, miR-222 could be a potential therapeutic target against cardiac stress.[75]

miRNAs have also been shown to be secreted into the bloodstream in response to exercise (referred to as circulating miRNAs [c-miRNAs]). Of interest, the regulation of c-miRNAs in humans seems to be influenced by exercise type, duration, and intensity of the training (eg, sustained aerobic, acute exhaustive, resistance, endurance).[82–87] Further studies will be required to determine whether these miRNAs play key roles in regulating exercise-induced cardiac remodeling.

Other Factors Affecting Exercise-induced Cardiac Remodeling

Although not the focus of this article, it is recognized that other factors, including genetic factors, epigenetics, sex, and diet can have an effect on molecular pathways and consequently how the heart responds to exercise training.[1,88,89] For instance, polymorphisms within genes, including angiotensin-converting enzyme and angiotensinogen, have been associated with greater cardiac enlargement in response to exercise training.[1,90] Polymorphisms in other genes that may affect exercise-induced cardiac remodeling include interleukin-17A (associated with reduced cardiac growth and high aerobic performance in skiers[91]), and NO synthase (NOS3; associated with greater RV enlargement in athletes participating in water sports[92]). Exercise can also induce epigenetic changes that are likely to contribute to remodeling. Although this has not been studied extensively in the heart, common exercise-induced epigenetic changes identified in a range of organs/systems include methylation and acetylation, DNA methylation, and altered expression of miRNAs.[89]

MOLECULAR MECHANISMS ASSOCIATED WITH MALADAPTIVE EXERCISE-INDUCED CARDIAC REMODELING

Cellular and molecular mechanisms responsible for maladaptive exercise-induced cardiac remodeling have been less studied and are not well defined. However, prolonged increase of catecholamine levels, reduced β-adrenergic sensitivity, and increased oxidative stress have been implicated as stimuli (see **Table 1**).[93,94] Of note, these stimuli are also common to cardiac disease settings in which there is dysregulation of G protein–coupled receptor signaling pathways and regulators that induce pathologic cardiac remodeling (eg, calcineurin).[4]

Models used to examine molecular mechanisms contributing to maladaptive exercise-induced remodeling are summarized in **Table 2**. A rat model of long-term, intensive endurance exercise (treadmill running for 16 weeks) was shown to be associated with diastolic and systolic dysfunction, and fibrosis within the RV.[95] The triggers mediating this response are not entirely clear, although it is possible that intensive exercise led to secretion of fibrogenic mediators (eg, tumor necrosis factor α [TNFα], TGFβ, and endothelin-1) from cardiac cells (eg, myocytes,

immune cells, and vascular cells) leading to cardiac fibrosis.[53] It is also noteworthy that the treadmill running protocol incorporated a small electric shock to ensure that running was maintained. Thus, the possibility cannot entirely be excluded that the exercise protocol also induced emotional stress.[95]

Another area of investigation has been related to strenuous exercise–induced atrial remodeling and arrhythmia; for example, atrial fibrillation (AF). Increased AF susceptibility has been reported in some elite athletes undertaking high-intensity endurance exercise, such as cross-country skiing.[96,97] Backx and colleagues[98] developed 2 mouse models of intense endurance exercise to simulate levels similar to those attained by elite athletes undertaking long-term endurance sports. Mice were subjected to swim training or treadmill running for 6 weeks with exercise levels that exceeded 70% of the maximal oxygen uptake (VO_2 max) for the duration of the exercise.[98] These training protocols did not lead to a significant increase in heart mass or ventricular dysfunction. However, exercise was associated with increased cardiac chamber dimensions, increased normalized atrial weight, atrial fibrosis, atrial inflammation, and increased susceptibility to AF. TNFα-dependent activation of nuclear factor κB (NFκB) and p38 mitogen–activated protein kinase (MAPK) was implicated as a potential mechanism. Exercise-induced atrial abnormalities were prevented in TNFα KO mice.[98]

THERAPEUTIC APPROACHES THAT TARGET KEY MECHANISMS RESPONSIBLE FOR EXERCISE-INDUCED ADAPTIVE CARDIAC REMODELING

The benefits of exercise or regular physical activity in humans on reducing cardiovascular disease risk and all-cause mortality are well recognized.[43,99–101] Exercise has also been shown to provide cardiac protection in several animal models, including myocardial infarction (MI), ischemia/reperfusion injury, pressure overload, and cardiomyopathy (dilated, hypertrophic, diabetic).[44,54,102] Furthermore, many of the benefits of exercise can be mimicked, at least in part, by administering factors released with exercise (eg, IGF1, HGF) or via the transgenic expression of genes that play key roles in exercise-induced remodeling (eg, IGF1/IGF1R, PI3K, Akt).[2,4,44] Consequently, many investigators have assessed the therapeutic potential of regulating mediators of exercise-induced adaptive remodeling with gene therapy, miRNA-based treatments, and small molecules (**Fig. 3**).

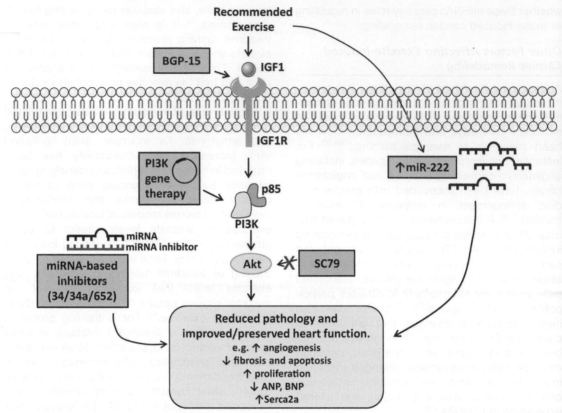

Fig. 3. Therapies targeting regulators of adaptive exercise-induced remodeling in a setting of cardiac stress, showing gene-based or small molecule–based therapies targeting adaptive processes of the heart that hold promise for the treatment of heart failure. BGP-15 and SC79 are small molecules that target IGF1R and Akt, respectively. SC79 did not provide cardiac protection (*red X*). Akt, protein kinase B; ANP, atrial natriuretic peptide; BNP, B-type natriuretic peptide; miRNA/miR, microRNA; SERCA2a, sarcoplasmic/endoplasmic reticulum Ca^{2+}-ATPase.

Gene Therapy

Having established that PI3K(p110α) is a critical mediator of exercise-induced cardiac hypertrophy and protection,[17,44] and that chronic activation of PI3K using a transgenic approach protects the heart in numerous cardiac disorders (MI,[77] pressure overload,[54] dilated cardiomyopathy,[54] AF,[55] diabetic cardiomyopathy[103]), Weeks and colleagues[44] proceeded to develop a gene therapy (recombinant adeno-associated virus [AAV]) to deliver PI3K(p110α) selectively to hearts of adult mice with established cardiac disorder.[44] Muscle-specific delivery of PI3K(p110α) was able to improve heart function in mice with established adverse remodeling caused by aortic banding.[44] More recently, another PI3K isoform (PI3K, p110β) was targeted with AAV9, which also selectively transduces the heart. Gene delivery of PI3K(p110β) promoted cardiac myocyte survival (proliferation and reduced apoptosis) in mice after MI.[104] Mechanisms implicated included regulation of Akt and p27.[104]

MicroRNA-based Treatments

Targeting miRNAs in preclinical models of cardiac disease has been promising,[105] and an miRNA-based therapy for hepatitis C (Miravirsen) was shown to be well tolerated and effective in a clinical trial.[106] Consequently, several miRNA-based drugs (eg, miRNA inhibitors; antisense oligonucleotides) are currently under development.[105] Investigators have begun exploring the potential of targeting miRNAs regulated in the heart in response to exercise (eg, miR-222) or those miRNAs regulated by key pathways responsible for exercise-induced cardiac remodeling (eg, PI3K).[80] As noted earlier, transgenic miR-222 mice were protected in a setting of ischemic injury; however, an approach to pharmacologically increase miR-222 levels is yet to be described.[75] Bernardo and colleagues have focused on PI3K-regulated miRNAs, namely the miR-34a/miR-34 family (miR-34a, miR-34b, miR-34c) and miR-652.[107–109] These miRNAs were distinctly regulated in settings of adaptive cardiac remodeling and cardiac disease; that is, expression was lower in protected hearts with increased PI3K(p110α) signaling but increased in diseased hearts caused by MI.[77] The administration of miRNA inhibitors against miR-34a/miR-34 family or miR-652 was associated with protection in cardiac injury models (MI and pressure overload; eg, better heart function, less fibrosis and apoptosis, increased angiogenesis, and improved molecular signature).[107–109] Other investigators have subsequently confirmed that silencing miR-34a in the diseased heart represents a promising approach.[110–112]

Small Molecules That Activate the Insulin-like Growth Factor 1–Phosphoinositide 3-Kinase–Protein Kinase B Signaling Cascade

Small molecule–activating insulin-like growth factor 1 receptor

Sapra and colleagues[120] examined the therapeutic potential of a small molecule (BGP-15) in a transgenic mouse model that develops heart failure and AF. BGP-15 is a hydroximic acid derivative that was previously shown to coinduce the stress-inducible form of heat shock protein 70 (Hsp70).[113–115] BGP-15 was an attractive drug to test in a preclinical model with a cardiac disorder because BGP-15 was not associated with any adverse cardiac events or other serious side effects in several clinical trials for other conditions (eg, diabetes).[116–119] Four weeks of BGP-15 treatment in the mouse model with heart failure and AF was associated with improved cardiac remodeling and function and reduced episodes of arrhythmia.[120] Note that BGP-15 phosphorylated the IGF1R rather than inducing Hsp70, and activation of IGF1R seems to be the mechanism via which BGP-15 mediates cardiac protection.[120]

Small molecule–activating protein kinase B

The therapeutic potential of a small molecule activator of Akt (SC79) was recently investigated in the heart in a setting of ischemia-reperfusion.[121] SC79 activated Akt within the heart; however, SC79 administered in low or high doses before or after ischemia did not inhibit apoptosis, rescue cardiac myocardium ATP levels, or affect the activity of mitochondrial enzymes. Furthermore, SC79 failed to reduce infarct size or the release of cardiac injury biomarkers at reperfusion. The conclusion from these experiments was that acute pharmacologic activation of Akt may not be sufficient to provide protection against ischemia.[121] Given that some mitochondrial adaptations in response to exercise have been shown to be PI3K dependent but Akt independent,[22] activation of Akt alone may be insufficient in this stress setting.

SUMMARY

Several key mediators of adaptive exercise-induced cardiac remodeling have been identified from animal studies. IGF1-PI3K signaling has been implicated as a critical regulator of many cellular responses that accompany adaptive exercise-induced remodeling, including cardiac myocyte hypertrophy, mitochondrial biogenesis, sarcomeric remodeling, electrical remodeling, and angiogenesis. Although still in the preclinical stages, targeting the IGF1-PI3K pathway in cardiac disease settings seems to represent a promising approach. However, despite significant progress in understanding the molecular mechanisms that accompany exercise-induced remodeling, further studies are required. To date, investigators have largely focused on examining molecular mechanisms responsible for adaptive exercise-induced heart growth within the LV or mixed ventricular tissue. Studies describing the molecular mechanisms responsible for maladaptive exercise-induced cardiac remodeling, as well as mechanisms within the RV and atria (under adaptive and maladaptive settings) are sparse in comparison.[93,122,123] Mechanisms governing how the RV and atria respond to exercise are likely to differ, which is particularly important given that prolonged endurance exercise may affect the RV and atria more than the LV.[6] In addition, the most common exercise models used in rodent studies (eg, swim training, voluntary free wheel or treadmill running) do not necessarily mimic all forms of exercise-induced cardiac remodeling in humans (eg, strength training). Molecular mechanisms are likely to differ based on the type of exercise, intensity, and duration. It is hoped that a more comprehensive understanding of the molecular basis of different forms of exercise-induced cardiac remodeling will result in the identification of additional molecular targets for pharmacologic intervention.

REFERENCES

1. Weiner RB, Baggish AL. Cardiovascular adaptation and remodeling to rigorous athletic training. Clin Sports Med 2015;34(3):405–18.
2. Wilson MG, Ellison GM, Cable NT. Basic science behind the cardiovascular benefits of exercise. Heart 2015;101(10):758–65.
3. Mihl C, Dassen WR, Kuipers H. Cardiac remodelling: concentric versus eccentric hypertrophy in strength and endurance athletes. Neth Heart J 2008;16(4):129–33.
4. Bernardo BC, Weeks KL, Pretorius L, et al. Molecular distinction between physiological and

pathological cardiac hypertrophy: experimental findings and therapeutic strategies. Pharmacol Ther 2010;128(1):191–227.

5. Tham YK, Bernardo BC, Ooi JY, et al. Pathophysiology of cardiac hypertrophy and heart failure: signaling pathways and novel therapeutic targets. Arch Toxicol 2015;89(9):1401–38.

6. La Gerche A, Heidbuchel H. Can intensive exercise harm the heart? You can get too much of a good thing. Circulation 2014; 130(12):992–1002.

7. Yasuda S, Goto Y, Takaki H, et al. Exercise-induced hepatocyte growth factor production in patients after acute myocardial infarction: its relationship to exercise capacity and brain natriuretic peptide levels. Circ J 2004;68(4):304–7.

8. Czarkowska-Paczek B, Bartlomiejczyk I, Przybylski J. The serum levels of growth factors: PDGF, TGF-beta and VEGF are increased after strenuous physical exercise. J Physiol Pharmacol 2006;57(2):189–97.

9. Porrello ER, Mahmoud AI, Simpson E, et al. Transient regenerative potential of the neonatal mouse heart. Science 2011;331(6020):1078–80.

10. Soonpaa MH, Field LJ. Survey of studies examining mammalian cardiomyocyte DNA synthesis. Circ Res 1998;83(1):15–26.

11. Soonpaa MH, Kim KK, Pajak L, et al. Cardiomyocyte DNA synthesis and binucleation during murine development. Am J Physiol 1996;271(5 Pt 2): H2183–9.

12. Leite CF, Lopes CS, Alves AC, et al. Endogenous resident c-Kit cardiac stem cells increase in mice with an exercise-induced, physiologically hypertrophied heart. Stem Cell Res 2015; 15(1):151–64.

13. Waring CD, Vicinanza C, Papalamprou A, et al. The adult heart responds to increased workload with physiologic hypertrophy, cardiac stem cell activation, and new myocyte formation. Eur Heart J 2014;35(39):2722–31.

14. Bostrom P, Mann N, Wu J, et al. C/EBPbeta controls exercise-induced cardiac growth and protects against pathological cardiac remodeling. Cell 2010;143(7):1072–83.

15. Conlon I, Raff M. Size control in animal development. Cell 1999;96(2):235–44.

16. Neri-Serneri GG, Boddi M, Modesti PA, et al. Increased cardiac sympathetic activity and insulin-like growth factor-I formation are associated with physiological hypertrophy in athletes. Circ Res 2001;89(11):977–82.

17. McMullen JR, Shioi T, Zhang L, et al. Phosphoinositide 3-kinase(p110alpha) plays a critical role for the induction of physiological, but not pathological, cardiac hypertrophy. Proc Natl Acad Sci U S A 2003;100(21):12355–60.

18. DeBosch B, Treskov I, Lupu TS, et al. Akt1 is required for physiological cardiac growth. Circulation 2006;113(17):2097–104.

19. Kim J, Wende AR, Sena S, et al. Insulin-like growth factor I receptor signaling is required for exercise-induced cardiac hypertrophy. Mol Endocrinol 2008; 22(11):2531–43.

20. Luo J, McMullen JR, Sobkiw CL, et al. Class IA phosphoinositide 3-kinase regulates heart size and physiological cardiac hypertrophy. Mol Cell Biol 2005;25(21):9491–502.

21. Noh J, Wende AR, Olsen CD, et al. Phosphoinositide dependent protein kinase 1 is required for exercise-induced cardiac hypertrophy but not the associated mitochondrial adaptations. J Mol Cell Cardiol 2015;89(Pt B):297–305.

22. O'Neill BT, Kim J, Wende AR, et al. A conserved role for phosphatidylinositol 3-kinase but not Akt signaling in mitochondrial adaptations that accompany physiological cardiac hypertrophy. Cell Metab 2007;6(4):294–306.

23. Mao K, Kobayashi S, Jaffer ZM, et al. Regulation of Akt/PKB activity by P21-activated kinase in cardiomyocytes. J Mol Cell Cardiol 2008;44(2):429–34.

24. Davis RT 3rd, Simon JN, Utter M, et al. Knockout of p21-activated kinase-1 attenuates exercise-induced cardiac remodelling through altered calcineurin signalling. Cardiovasc Res 2015;108(3): 335–47.

25. Volkers M, Toko H, Doroudgar S, et al. Pathological hypertrophy amelioration by PRAS40-mediated inhibition of mTORC1. Proc Natl Acad Sci U S A 2013;110(31):12661–6.

26. McMullen JR, Shioi T, Huang W-Y, et al. The insulin-like growth factor 1 receptor induces physiological heart growth via the phosphoinositide 3-kinase (p110alpha) pathway. J Biol Chem 2004;279(6): 4782–93.

27. Moc C, Taylor AE, Chesini GP, et al. Physiological activation of Akt by PHLPP1 deletion protects against pathological hypertrophy. Cardiovasc Res 2015;105(2):160–70.

28. McMullen JR, Shioi T, Zhang L, et al. Deletion of ribosomal S6 kinases does not attenuate pathological, physiological, or insulin-like growth factor 1 receptor-phosphoinositide 3-kinase-induced cardiac hypertrophy. Mol Cell Biol 2004;24(14): 6231–40.

29. Wideman L, Weltman JY, Hartman ML, et al. Growth hormone release during acute and chronic aerobic and resistance exercise: recent findings. Sports Med 2002;32(15):987–1004.

30. Odiete O, Hill MF, Sawyer DB. Neuregulin in cardiovascular development and disease. Circ Res 2012; 111(10):1376–85.

31. Isgaard J, Wahlander H, Adams MA, et al. Increased expression of growth hormone receptor

mRNA and insulin-like growth factor-I mRNA in volume-overloaded hearts. Hypertension 1994; 23(6 Pt 2):884–8.

32. Bruel A, Christoffersen TE, Nyengaard JR. Growth hormone increases the proliferation of existing cardiac myocytes and the total number of cardiac myocytes in the rat heart. Cardiovasc Res 2007;76(3): 400–8.

33. Chintalgattu V, Ai D, Langley RR, et al. Cardiomyocyte PDGFR-beta signaling is an essential component of the mouse cardiac response to load-induced stress. J Clin Invest 2010;120(2):472–84.

34. Mellor HR, Bell AR, Valentin JP, et al. Cardiotoxicity associated with targeting kinase pathways in cancer. Toxicol Sci 2011;120(1):14–32.

35. Joseph-Bravo P, Jaimes-Hoy L, Uribe RM, et al. 60 years of neuroendocrinology: TRH, the first hypophysiotropic releasing hormone isolated: control of the pituitary-thyroid axis. J Endocrinol 2015; 226(2):T85–100.

36. Arechederra M, Carmona R, Gonzalez-Nunez M, et al. Met signaling in cardiomyocytes is required for normal cardiac function in adult mice. Biochim Biophys Acta 2013;1832(12):2204–15.

37. Bergmann O, Bhardwaj RD, Bernard S, et al. Evidence for cardiomyocyte renewal in humans. Science 2009;324(5923):98–102.

38. Senyo SE, Steinhauser ML, Pizzimenti CL, et al. Mammalian heart renewal by pre-existing cardiomyocytes. Nature 2013;493(7432):433–6.

39. Xiao J, Xu T, Li J, et al. Exercise-induced physiological hypertrophy initiates activation of cardiac progenitor cells. Int J Clin Exp Pathol 2014;7(2): 663–9.

40. Siu PM, Bryner RW, Martyn JK, et al. Apoptotic adaptations from exercise training in skeletal and cardiac muscles. FASEB J 2004;18(10):1150–2.

41. Jin H, Yang R, Li W, et al. Effects of exercise training on cardiac function, gene expression, and apoptosis in rats. Am J Physiol Heart Circ Physiol 2000;279(6):H2994–3002.

42. Werner C, Hanhoun M, Widmann T, et al. Effects of physical exercise on myocardial telomere-regulating proteins, survival pathways, and apoptosis. J Am Coll Cardiol 2008;52(6):470–82.

43. Wei X, Liu X, Rosenzweig A. What do we know about the cardiac benefits of exercise? Trends Cardiovasc Med 2015;25(6):529–36.

44. Weeks KL, Gao X, Du XJ, et al. Phosphoinositide 3-kinase p110alpha is a master regulator of exercise-induced cardioprotection and PI3K gene therapy rescues cardiac dysfunction. Circ Heart Fail 2012; 5(4):523–34.

45. Oka T, Maillet M, Watt AJ, et al. Cardiac-specific deletion of Gata4 reveals its requirement for hypertrophy, compensation, and myocyte viability. Circ Res 2006;98(6):837–45.

46. Bisping E, Ikeda S, Sedej M, et al. Transcription factor GATA4 is activated but not required for insulin-like growth factor 1 (IGF1)-induced cardiac hypertrophy. J Biol Chem 2012;287(13):9827–34.

47. Sakamoto M, Minamino T, Toko H, et al. Upregulation of heat shock transcription factor 1 plays a critical role in adaptive cardiac hypertrophy. Circ Res 2006;99(12):1411–8.

48. Kemi OJ, Wisloff U. Mechanisms of exercise-induced improvements in the contractile apparatus of the mammalian myocardium. Acta Physiol 2010; 199(4):425–39.

49. Moore RL, Palmer BM. Exercise training and cellular adaptations of normal and diseased hearts. Exerc Sport Sci Rev 1999;27:285–315.

50. Shan J, Kushnir A, Betzenhauser MJ, et al. Phosphorylation of the ryanodine receptor mediates the cardiac fight or flight response in mice. J Clin Invest 2010;120(12):4388–98.

51. Rohrer DK, Schauble EH, Desai KH, et al. Alterations in dynamic heart rate control in the beta 1-adrenergic receptor knockout mouse. Am J Physiol 1998;274(4 Pt 2):H1184–93.

52. Waardenberg AJ, Bernardo BC, Ng DC, et al. Phosphoinositide 3-kinase (PI3K(p110alpha)) directly regulates key components of the Z-disc and cardiac structure. J Biol Chem 2011;286(35): 30837–46.

53. Martin ML, Blaxall BC. Cardiac intercellular communication: are myocytes and fibroblasts fair-weather friends? J Cardiovasc Transl Res 2012; 5(6):768–82.

54. McMullen JR, Amirahmadi F, Woodcock EA, et al. Protective effects of exercise and phosphoinositide 3-kinase(p110alpha) signaling in dilated and hypertrophic cardiomyopathy. Proc Natl Acad Sci U S A 2007;104(2):612–7.

55. Pretorius L, Du XJ, Woodcock EA, et al. Reduced phosphoinositide 3-kinase (p110alpha) activation increases the susceptibility to atrial fibrillation. Am J Pathol 2009;175(3):998–1009.

56. Stanley WC, Chandler MP. Energy metabolism in the normal and failing heart: potential for therapeutic interventions. Heart Fail Rev 2002;7(2): 115–30.

57. Dobrzyn P, Pyrkowska A, Duda MK, et al. Expression of lipogenic genes is upregulated in the heart with exercise training-induced but not pressure overload-induced left ventricular hypertrophy. Am J Physiol Endocrinol Metab 2013; 304(12):E1348–58.

58. Ohkuwa T, Sato Y, Naoi M. Glutathione status and reactive oxygen generation in tissues of young and old exercised rats. Acta Physiol Scand 1997; 159(3):237–44.

59. Richters L, Lange N, Renner R, et al. Exercise-induced adaptations of cardiac redox homeostasis

and remodeling in heterozygous SOD2-knockout mice. J Appl Physiol (1985) 2011;111(5):1431–40.

60. Powers SK, Sollanek KJ, Wiggs MP, et al. Exercise-induced improvements in myocardial antioxidant capacity: the antioxidant players and cardioprotection. Free Radic Res 2014;48(1):43–51.

61. Yang KC, Foeger NC, Marionneau C, et al. Homeostatic regulation of electrical excitability in physiological cardiac hypertrophy. J Physiol 2010;588(Pt 24):5015–32.

62. Brown MD. Exercise and coronary vascular remodelling in the healthy heart. Exp Physiol 2003;88(5):645–58.

63. White FC, Bloor CM, McKirnan MD, et al. Exercise training in swine promotes growth of arteriolar bed and capillary angiogenesis in heart. J Appl Physiol (1985) 1998;85(3):1160–8.

64. Bekhite MM, Finkensieper A, Binas S, et al. VEGF-mediated PI3K class IA and PKC signaling in cardiomyogenesis and vasculogenesis of mouse embryonic stem cells. J Cell Sci 2011;124(Pt 11):1819–30.

65. Olfert IM, Howlett RA, Tang K, et al. Muscle-specific VEGF deficiency greatly reduces exercise endurance in mice. J Physiol 2009;587(Pt 8):1755–67.

66. Shiojima I, Sato K, Izumiya Y, et al. Disruption of coordinated cardiac hypertrophy and angiogenesis contributes to the transition to heart failure. J Clin Invest 2005;115(8):2108–18.

67. Dimmeler S, Assmus B, Hermann C, et al. Fluid shear stress stimulates phosphorylation of Akt in human endothelial cells: involvement in suppression of apoptosis. Circ Res 1998;83(3):334–41.

68. Dimmeler S, Fleming I, Fisslthaler B, et al. Activation of nitric oxide synthase in endothelial cells by Akt-dependent phosphorylation. Nature 1999;399(6736):601–5.

69. Calvert JW, Condit ME, Aragon JP, et al. Exercise protects against myocardial ischemia-reperfusion injury via stimulation of beta(3)-adrenergic receptors and increased nitric oxide signaling: role of nitrite and nitrosothiols. Circ Res 2011;108(12):1448–58.

70. Hata A. Functions of microRNAs in cardiovascular biology and disease. Annu Rev Physiol 2013;75:69–93.

71. Small EM, Olson EN. Pervasive roles of microRNAs in cardiovascular biology. Nature 2011;469(7330):336–42.

72. Martinelli NC, Cohen CR, Santos KG, et al. An analysis of the global expression of microRNAs in an experimental model of physiological left ventricular hypertrophy. PLoS One 2014;9(4):e93271.

73. Fernandes T, Barauna VG, Negrao CE, et al. Aerobic exercise training promotes physiological cardiac remodeling involving a set of microRNAs.

74. Fernandes T, Hashimoto NY, Magalhaes FC, et al. Aerobic exercise training-induced left ventricular hypertrophy involves regulatory microRNAs, decreased angiotensin-converting enzyme-angiotensin II, and synergistic regulation of angiotensin-converting enzyme 2-angiotensin (1-7). Hypertension 2011;58(2):182–9.

75. Liu X, Xiao J, Zhu H, et al. miR-222 is necessary for exercise-induced cardiac growth and protects against pathological cardiac remodeling. Cell Metab 2015;21(4):584–95.

76. Ma Z, Qi J, Meng S, et al. Swimming exercise training-induced left ventricular hypertrophy involves microRNAs and synergistic regulation of the PI3K/AKT/mTOR signaling pathway. Eur J Appl Physiol 2013;113(10):2473–86.

77. Lin RC, Weeks KL, Gao XM, et al. PI3K(p110 alpha) protects against myocardial infarction-induced heart failure: identification of PI3K-regulated miRNA and mRNA. Arterioscler Thromb Vasc Biol 2010;30(4):724–32.

78. Care A, Catalucci D, Felicetti F, et al. MicroRNA-133 controls cardiac hypertrophy. Nat Med 2007;13(5):613–8.

79. Soci UP, Fernandes T, Hashimoto NY, et al. MicroRNAs 29 are involved in the improvement of ventricular compliance promoted by aerobic exercise training in rats. Physiol Genomics 2011;43(11):665–73.

80. Ooi JY, Bernardo BC, McMullen JR. The therapeutic potential of miRNAs regulated in settings of physiological cardiac hypertrophy. Future Med Chem 2014;6(2):205–22.

81. Mann N, Rosenzweig A. Can exercise teach us how to treat heart disease? Circulation 2012;126(22):2625–35.

82. Baggish AL, Hale A, Weiner RB, et al. Dynamic regulation of circulating microRNA during acute exhaustive exercise and sustained aerobic exercise training. J Physiol 2011;589(Pt 16):3983–94.

83. Sawada S, Kon M, Wada S, et al. Profiling of circulating microRNAs after a bout of acute resistance exercise in humans. PLoS One 2013;8(7):e70823.

84. Mooren FC, Viereck J, Kruger K, et al. Circulating microRNAs as potential biomarkers of aerobic exercise capacity. Am J Physiol Heart Circ Physiol 2014;306(4):H557–63.

85. Baggish AL, Park J, Min PK, et al. Rapid upregulation and clearance of distinct circulating microRNAs after prolonged aerobic exercise. J Appl Physiol (1985) 2014;116(5):522–31.

86. Banzet S, Chennaoui M, Girard O, et al. Changes in circulating microRNAs levels with exercise modality. J Appl Physiol (1985) 2013;115(9):1237–44.

Am J Physiol Heart Circ Physiol 2015;309(4):H543–52.

87. de Gonzalo-Calvo D, Davalos A, Montero A, et al. Circulating inflammatory miRNA signature in response to different doses of aerobic exercise. J Appl Physiol (1985) 2015;119(2):124–34.

88. Konhilas JP, Chen H, Luczak E, et al. Diet and sex modify exercise and cardiac adaptation in the mouse. Am J Physiol Heart Circ Physiol 2015; 308(2):H135–45.

89. Ntanasis-Stathopoulos J, Tzanninis JG, Philippou A, et al. Epigenetic regulation on gene expression induced by physical exercise. J Musculoskelet Neuronal Interact 2013;13(2):133–46.

90. Pelliccia A, Thompson PD. The genetics of left ventricular remodeling in competitive athletes. J Cardiovasc Med (Hagerstown) 2006;7(4):267–70.

91. Lifanov AD, Khadyeva MN, Demenev SV, et al. Association of G197 polymorphism of IL-17A gene with myocardial remodeling and aerobic performance in athletes. Bull Exp Biol Med 2014;157(5): 659–62.

92. Szelid Z, Lux A, Kolossvary M, et al. Right ventricular adaptation is associated with the Glu298Asp variant of the NOS3 gene in elite athletes. PLoS One 2015;10(10):e0141680.

93. Eijsvogels TM, Fernandez AB, Thompson PD. Are there deleterious cardiac effects of acute and chronic endurance exercise? Physiol Rev 2016; 96(1):99–125.

94. Gielen S, Schuler G, Adams V. Cardiovascular effects of exercise training: molecular mechanisms. Circulation 2010;122(12):1221–38.

95. Benito B, Gay-Jordi G, Serrano-Mollar A, et al. Cardiac arrhythmogenic remodeling in a rat model of long-term intensive exercise training. Circulation 2011;123(1):13–22.

96. Grimsmo J, Grundvold I, Maehlum S, et al. High prevalence of atrial fibrillation in long-term endurance cross-country skiers: echocardiographic findings and possible predictors–a 28-30 years follow-up study. Eur J Cardiovasc Prev Rehabil 2010;17(1):100–5.

97. Andersen K, Farahmand B, Ahlbom A, et al. Risk of arrhythmias in 52 755 long-distance cross-country skiers: a cohort study. Eur Heart J 2013;34(47): 3624–31.

98. Aschar-Sobbi R, Izaddoustdar F, Korogyi AS, et al. Increased atrial arrhythmia susceptibility induced by intense endurance exercise in mice requires TNFalpha. Nat Commun 2015;6: 6018.

99. Blair SN, Kohl HW 3rd, Paffenbarger RS Jr, et al. Physical fitness and all-cause mortality. A prospective study of healthy men and women. JAMA 1989; 262(17):2395–401.

100. Kodama S, Saito K, Tanaka S, et al. Cardiorespiratory fitness as a quantitative predictor of all-cause mortality and cardiovascular events in healthy men and women: a meta-analysis. JAMA 2009; 301(19):2024–35.

101. Lee DC, Sui X, Artero EG, et al. Long-term effects of changes in cardiorespiratory fitness and body mass index on all-cause and cardiovascular disease mortality in men: the Aerobics Center Longitudinal Study. Circulation 2011;124(23):2483–90.

102. Tao L, Bei Y, Zhang H, et al. Exercise for the heart: signaling pathways. Oncotarget 2015;6(25): 20773–84.

103. Ritchie RH, Love JE, Huynh K, et al. Enhanced phosphoinositide 3-kinase(p110alpha) activity prevents diabetes-induced cardiomyopathy and superoxide generation in a mouse model of diabetes. Diabetologia 2012;55(12):3369–81.

104. Lin Z, Zhou P, von Gise A, et al. Pi3kcb links Hippo-YAP and PI3K-AKT signaling pathways to promote cardiomyocyte proliferation and survival. Circ Res 2015;116(1):35–45.

105. Bernardo BC, Ooi JY, Lin RC, et al. miRNA therapeutics: a new class of drugs with potential therapeutic applications in the heart. Future Med Chem 2015;7(13):1771–92.

106. Janssen HL, Reesink HW, Lawitz EJ, et al. Treatment of HCV infection by targeting microRNA. N Engl J Med 2013;368(18):1685–94.

107. Bernardo BC, Gao XM, Tham YK, et al. Silencing of miR-34a attenuates cardiac dysfunction in a setting of moderate, but not severe, hypertrophic cardiomyopathy. PLoS One 2014;9(2):e90337.

108. Bernardo BC, Gao XM, Winbanks CE, et al. Therapeutic inhibition of the miR-34 family attenuates pathological cardiac remodeling and improves heart function. Proc Natl Acad Sci U S A 2012; 109(43):17615–20.

109. Bernardo BC, Nguyen SS, Winbanks CE, et al. Therapeutic silencing of miR-652 restores heart function and attenuates adverse remodeling in a setting of established pathological hypertrophy. FASEB J 2014;28(12):5097–110.

110. Boon RA, Iekushi K, Lechner S, et al. MicroRNA-34a regulates cardiac ageing and function. Nature 2013;495(7439):107–10.

111. Huang Y, Qi Y, Du JQ, et al. MicroRNA-34a regulates cardiac fibrosis after myocardial infarction by targeting Smad4. Expert Opin Ther Targets 2014;18(12):1355–65.

112. Yang Y, Cheng HW, Qiu Y, et al. MicroRNA-34a plays a key role in cardiac repair and regeneration following myocardial infarction. Circ Res 2015; 117(5):450–9.

113. Chung J, Nguyen A-K, Henstridge DC, et al. HSP72 protects against obesity-induced insulin resistance. Proc Natl Acad Sci U S A 2008; 105(5):1739–44.

114. Gehrig SM, van der Poel C, Sayer TA, et al. Hsp72 preserves muscle function and slows progression

of severe muscular dystrophy. Nature 2012; 484(7394):394–8.

115. Crul T, Toth N, Piotto S, et al. Hydroximic acid derivatives: pleiotropic HSP co-inducers restoring homeostasis and robustness. Curr Pharm Des 2013; 19(3):309–46.

116. Literati-Nagy B, Kulcsar E, Literati-Nagy Z, et al. Improvement of insulin sensitivity by a novel drug, BGP-15, in insulin-resistant patients: a proof of concept randomized double-blind clinical trial. Horm Metab Res 2009;41(5):374–80.

117. Literati-Nagy B, Peterfai E, Kulcsar E, et al. Beneficial effect of the insulin sensitizer (HSP inducer) BGP-15 on olanzapine-induced metabolic disorders. Brain Res Bull 2010;83(6): 340–4.

118. Literati-Nagy Z, Tory K, Literati-Nagy B, et al. The HSP co-inducer BGP-15 can prevent the metabolic side effects of the atypical antipsychotics. Cell Stress Chaperones 2012;17(4):517–21.

119. Febbraio MA. Role of chemical chaperones in treatment for type 2 diabetes. Proceedings of the IDF World Diabetes Congress. Melbourne, December 2–6, 2013.

120. Sapra G, Tham YK, Cemerlang N, et al. The small-molecule BGP-15 protects against heart failure and atrial fibrillation in mice. Nat Commun 2014;5:5705.

121. Moreira JB, Wohlwend M, Alves MN, et al. A small molecule activator of AKT does not reduce ischemic injury of the rat heart. J Transl Med 2015;13:76.

122. Poels EM, da Costa Martins PA, van Empel VP. Adaptive capacity of the right ventricle: why does it fail? Am J Physiol Heart Circ Physiol 2015; 308(8):H803–13.

123. Voelkel NF, Quaife RA, Leinwand LA, et al. Right ventricular function and failure: report of a National Heart, Lung, and Blood Institute working group on cellular and molecular mechanisms of right heart failure. Circulation 2006;114(17):1883–91.

Sudden Cardiac Death in Athletes: Still Much to Learn

Joanna Sweeting, BSc, MAppSci (Env. Sci)[a,b],
Christopher Semsarian, MBBS, PhD, MPH, FRACP, FHRS, FCSANZ[a,b,c,*]

KEYWORDS

• Sudden cardiac death • Athletes • Genetics

KEY POINTS

• Sudden cardiac death (SCD) in athletes is a rare but tragic event with an incidence of approximately 1 in 50,000.
• Common causes of SCD in athletes include the structural and arrhythmogenic genetic heart diseases, which are inherited as autosomal dominant traits.
• The process following an SCD in an athlete involves a comprehensive postmortem examination, clinical family screening, and genetic testing.
• It is vitally important to identify, where possible, the cause of death in these cases. If a genetic heart disease is suspected, family members should be thoroughly examined to identify other individuals with disease who are therefore at risk of SCD.
• Many questions remain unanswered, including differences in the causes of SCD in athletes globally, and establishing the best approaches to identify those athletes at highest risk of SCD.

INTRODUCTION

The sudden cardiac death (SCD) of any individual is a tragic event, particularly when there has been no sign of disease before death. In athletes, the impact may be felt more acutely because these individuals are often young and widely thought to be the epitome of health and fitness.[1] This perception is often exploited in media coverage of SCD, further amplifying the impact of these tragedies, not just for the family of the individual but for the entire community.[2,3] Because of the emotive nature of these events, it is imperative that those who encounter the individuals and families affected by these tragedies are well informed of the potential causes and course of action required following an SCD.

To be classified as an SCD, the death must occur within 1 hour from the onset of symptoms in witnessed cases, and within 24 hours of the individual last being seen alive and well in unwitnessed cases.[4] In athletes, SCD can occur at any time during competition, in training, or even occasionally at rest.[5] Other possible causes, such as respiratory, cerebrovascular, and drug-related causes, must be excluded. An athlete may be defined as an individual who engages in regular, intense physical activity through competition and training, with an emphasis on striving to improve and achieve.[6] This definition encompasses paid professional sportspersons as well as university, college, and high school students, and may be extended to include children and adolescents involved in organized sporting activities. Competitive athletes include those who exercise for more than 10 hours per week, whereas those engaged in sports for recreational activities usually participate for less than 10 hours per week.[7]

a Agnes Ginges Centre for Molecular Cardiology, Centenary Institute, Locked Bag 6, Newtown, New South Wales 2042, Australia; b Sydney Medical School, Edward Ford Building, Fisher Road, University of Sydney, New South Wales 2006, Australia; c Department of Cardiology, Royal Prince Alfred Hospital, Missenden Road, Camperdown, New South Wales 2050, Australia
* Corresponding author. Agnes Ginges Centre for Molecular Cardiology, Centenary Institute, Locked Bag 6, Newtown, New South Wales 2042, Australia.
E-mail address: c.semsarian@centenary.org.au

Cardiol Clin 34 (2016) 531–541
http://dx.doi.org/10.1016/j.ccl.2016.06.003
0733-8651/16/© 2016 Elsevier Inc. All rights reserved.

This article briefly summarizes the current literature regarding the incidence of SCD in athletes and the possible underlying causes, with a focus on inherited heart diseases. The course of action following an SCD is discussed with respect to the postmortem examination; genetic testing, such as a molecular autopsy; and the implications for family members, including clinical and genetic screening. In addition, the areas in which there is still much to learn are discussed, including the difficulties associated with postmortem examination and genetic testing in these individuals, and the issue of divergence in the most common causes of SCD in athletes identified in different countries.

INCIDENCE OF SUDDEN CARDIAC DEATH IN ATHLETES

SCD is the most common medical cause of death among athletes, with a wide range of incidence rates reported; from 1 per 3000 to 1 per 917,000, depending on ethnicity and type of sport.[8] A large proportion of available incidence data comes from studies of athletes in the United States, both at high school and college level. A recent article from Harmon and colleagues[9] reported results from a study of 10 years of data from the National Collegiate Athletic Association (NCAA) in the United States. SCD accounted for 79 out of 514 deaths (~1 per 54,000 athlete years) over the 10-year period, with the incidence in men 3.2 times that of women.[9] Basketball players in general were found to have the highest risk of SCD, for both men and women, with a rate of ~1 per 15,000 athlete years. For men participating in division 1 basketball, the incidence increased to 1 per 5200 athlete years.[9] Black athletes were also found to be at higher risk of SCD than white athletes, with a rate of 1 per 21,491 athlete years compared with 1 per 68,354 athlete years. Another study, combining data from the NCAA database and the US National Registry of Sudden Death in Athletes database, found that 64 of 182 sudden deaths (35%) had cardiovascular causes and that cardiovascular deaths were 5 times more common in African American athletes than in white athletes over a period of 10 years.[10] This finding translates to an incidence of 1.2 per 100,000 athlete years, with black athletes again found to have a higher risk of SCD.

Elsewhere in the world similar studies have been conducted in an attempt to establish the incidence of SCD in athletes. A 7-year retrospective study in Denmark, of athletes aged 12 to 35 years, found an incidence rate of 1.2 per 100,000 athlete years or 1 per 82,645 sports-related SCDs in this specific age range.[11] A second retrospective study from Denmark incorporating data from a 3-year period showed a difference in the rate of SCD in athletes depending on age, with a rate of 0.47 per 100,000 athlete years in those aged 12 to 35 years and a rate of 6.64 per 100,000 athlete years for those aged 36 to 49 years.[12] This study also showed that incidence rates in competitive and noncompetitive or recreational athletes were similar and that the rate of SCD in the general population (10.7 per 100,000 person years) was much higher than sports-related SCD. A prospective study in Italy from 1979 to 1999 assessed rates of sudden death in athletes in the same age range of 12 to 35 years.[13] In athletes, the rate of SCD by cardiovascular causes was 2.1 per 100,000 athletes per year, giving an incidence of 1 per 47,600.

There are challenges in determining the true incidence of SCD in athletes because of differences in rates according to age, ethnicity, and chosen sport. Difficulties are also encountered in determining an accurate denominator for calculations and ensuring accurate reporting of sudden death events on databases and through the media.[8] Taking this into account, and based on the worldwide data from these and other retrospective and prospective studies, it is generally accepted that the incidence of SCD in athletes is within the range of 1 to 3 per 100,000, with the rate in the comprehensively studied cohort of NCAA athletes approximately 1 per 50,000.[9,14] Tragically, in many of these cases the first sign of disease is the SCD event, with a limited number of individuals aware of a preexisting heart condition.

CAUSES OF SUDDEN CARDIAC DEATH IN ATHLETES

The causes of SCD in athletes can be dichotomized into acquired and genetic causes. Acquired causes of SCD in athletes include myocarditis and coronary artery disease, in addition to those with external causes such as commotio cordis and drug misuse. In individuals 35 years of age and older, the most commonly identified cause of an SCD event is coronary artery disease, whereas for those aged less than 35 years the genetic heart diseases are more common.[1] The genetic conditions include structural diseases such as hypertrophic cardiomyopathy (HCM) and arrhythmogenic right ventricular cardiomyopathy/dysplasia (ARVC), and arrhythmogenic disorders including long QT syndrome (LQTS) and catecholaminergic polymorphic ventricular tachycardia (CPVT). A summary of the major features of these and other genetic heart diseases is shown in **Table 1**. In all these diseases, high-intensity and competitive physical activity is thought to increase the risk of

Table 1
Characteristics of common genetic heart diseases that may cause SCD in athletes

Genetic Heart Disease	Common Disease Genes	Symptoms	ECG/Echocardiogram Signs	Evidence of Disease at PM
Structural				
HCM	*MYBPC3, MYH7, TNNI3, TNNT2*	Chest pain, dyspnea, fatigue, syncope, palpitations	ECG: T-wave inversion Echocardiogram: LV wall thickening	Myocyte disarray, increased myocyte size, interstitial fibrosis
Arrhythmogenic right ventricular tachycardia	*DSC2, DSG2, DSP, PKP2, RYR2*	Palpitations, dizziness, syncope	ECG: Depolarization/ repolarization irregularities Echocardiogram: dilatation of RV ejection fraction, localized RV aneurysms	Myocardial atrophy, fibrofatty replacement of RV myocardium
Arrhythmogenic				
Long QT syndrome	*KCNQ1, KCNH2, SCN5a*	Syncope, fainting	ECG: prolonged QT interval	No evidence of disease
CPVT	*RYR2, CASQ2*	Emotional or stress-induced syncope	Ventricular arrhythmias on 24-h ECG Holter or during exercise stress test	No evidence of disease
Brugada syndrome	*CACNA1C, CACNA2D1, CACNB2, SCN5A, TRPM4*	Syncope caused by ventricular tachycardia or ventricular fibrillation	ECG: atypical right bundle branch block, cove-shaped ST elevation in leads V_1 to V_3	No evidence of disease
Wolff-Parkinson-White syndrome[a]	*PRKAG2*	Possible palpitations	ECG – bundle branch block, short PR interval, bouts of tachycardia	See note

Abbreviations: ECG, electrocardiogram; LV, left ventricle; PM, postmortem; RV, right ventricle.
[a] Wolff-Parkinson-White syndrome is a complex condition with potential for crossover with cardiomyopathy, with some individuals showing hypertrophy of the LV wall. Sporadic cases of Wolff-Parkinson-White do not generally have a familial basis. Individuals with PRKAG2 mutations generally have a combination of preexcitation and progressive atrioventricular conduction block.
Data from Refs.[27,35,40,58–61]

SCD through triggering of malignant ventricular arrhythmias.[15] These arrhythmias are induced by the physiologic changes occurring during exercise, such as altered catecholamine levels, acidosis, dehydration, and electrolyte imbalance.[16]

The genetic heart diseases are an important cause to be aware of in the context of SCD because these conditions are inherited as autosomal dominant traits, meaning that family members of affected individuals have a 1 in 2 chance of also carrying the disease-causing gene and being at increased risk of SCD.[17] For athletes who are diagnosed with a genetic heart disease while living, there are recommendations for physical activity after diagnosis.[18,19] In general, for both the structural and arrhythmogenic diseases, the recommendations include restriction from participation in competitive sports, apart from those of low intensity, such as golf, bowling, or yoga.[18,19] In some cases of arrhythmogenic disorders, such as LQTS, return to sport may be considered if treatment has been effective and appropriate precautionary measures have been taken.[18]

Inherited Structural Diseases

Hypertrophic cardiomyopathy
HCM is characterized by the presence of left ventricular wall thickening (in the absence of other loading conditions, such as hypertension).[20] It is a clinically heterogeneous disease in that patients may present with a range of symptoms, including dyspnea, fatigue, syncope, and chest pain, or no symptoms at all.[21] Individuals with HCM are also at an increased risk of SCD; a risk further heightened by high-intensity physical activity.[15] HCM is the most common inherited heart condition, with a prevalence of up to 1 per 200 in the general population.[22] HCM is therefore one of the most common causes of SCD in athletes in both the United States and the United Kingdom.[5,23]

Clinical signs of HCM indicating need for confirmatory echocardiogram include a heart murmur, a family history of HCM, unexplained syncope, and an abnormal electrocardiogram (ECG) pattern.[20] Abnormal ECG patterns are identified in approximately 90% of individuals with HCM and include T-wave inversion, ST segment depression, pathologic Q waves, conduction delay, left axis deviation, and left atrial enlargement.[24]

Arrhythmogenic right ventricular cardiomyopathy/dysplasia
ARVC, or previously arrhythmogenic right ventricular dysplasia, is another inherited cardiomyopathy that may cause SCD. The distinguishing feature of ARVC is myocyte loss with fibrofatty replacement primarily in the right ventricular myocardium,

although the left ventricle is also involved in up to 50% of cases.[25] It has a much lower prevalence compared with HCM at 1 per 5000 people, and most individuals with ARVC present after age 12 years, with symptoms including heart palpitations, dizziness, and syncope.[25] As with HCM, ARVC can also cause SCD and in some individuals, including athletes, this is the first sign of disease. Clinically, ARVC is diagnosed based on fulfillment of major and minor criteria, including abnormalities in the right ventricle on echocardiogram and depolarization/repolarization irregularities on ECG.[25]

Inherited Arrhythmia Disorders

The inherited arrhythmia disorders, also known as cardiac channelopathies, differ from the structural causes in that there are no macroscopic changes in the heart, both clinically and at postmortem, making diagnosis potentially more difficult. Although both have a much lower prevalence than HCM, LQTS (1 per 2000)[26] and CPVT (1 per 10,000)[27] are important causes to be aware of in the context of an SCD event. Other arrhythmogenic disorders include Brugada syndrome and Wolff-Parkinson-White syndrome, both of which can induce ventricular arrhythmias leading to SCD.

Long QT syndrome
Familial LQTS is an ion channelopathy that can lead to ventricular arrhythmias and SCD.[28] As with HCM and ARVC, individuals with LQTS may have no symptoms, or may experience symptoms such as syncope or near syncope.[29] Diagnosis is made clinically, most often on observation of a QTc between 480 and 499 milliseconds in multiple ECGs in the absence of a secondary cause, such as ingestion of QT-prolonging drugs.[29] LQTS can cause SCD because of abnormalities with depolarization and/or repolarization leading to the prolongation of the QT interval, which can degenerate into a ventricular tachycardia called torsades de pointes, ventricular fibrillation, and cardiac arrest. In athletes, swimming is a trigger, particularly in those with LQTS type 1.[30]

Catecholaminergic polymorphic ventricular tachycardia
Although one of the less common genetic heart diseases, CPVT is one of the most severe, with exercise and emotional stress triggers for cardiac arrest.[27] CPVT can present with emotional or physical stress–induced syncope at a young age, with the mean age of onset at age 7 to 9 years, in contrast with the structural disorders such as HCM that usually present in the second and third decades of life.[27] There are often no signs of disease on physical examination, ECG, and echocardiogram, with the

diagnosis of CPVT made by the identification of bidirectional ventricular tachycardia during an exercise test or on 24-hour ambulatory ECG monitoring.[27] A point of similarity between CPVT and other genetic heart diseases is the possibility that a SCD may be the first sign of disease.

Acquired Causes of Sudden Cardiac Death

Other potential causes of SCD in athletes in which the heart is structurally affected but may not have a definitive genetic basis include coronary artery disease and myocarditis, with both identified in numerous studies of athlete populations.[5,10,23,31] Further acquired causes of SCD in athletes include commotio cordis, which results from a blunt force trauma to the chest, eliciting ventricular fibrillation and cardiac arrest[32]; and drug misuse (including performance-enhancing drugs).[2]

WHEN TRAGEDY STRIKES: FOLLOWING THE SUDDEN CARDIAC DEATH OF AN ATHLETE

In most cases of SCD in the young (<40 years old), be it in an athlete or not, a postmortem examination is conducted. In Australia, consensus guidelines have been developed to ensure that all cases of SCD in the young are examined and a postmortem conducted to establish the cause of disease where possible.[33] This process is important not only in terms of finding an answer for why a young, fit, and seemingly healthy individual has died suddenly but also to determine whether a genetic heart disease was responsible and therefore whether family members may be at risk. There are 3 primary avenues of investigation following an SCD: postmortem examination, family screening, and genetic testing, as shown in the flow diagrams in **Figs. 1** and **2**.

Comprehensive Postmortem Examination

In most cases of sudden death in an athlete, a postmortem is conducted because these are generally unexpected events in individuals previously in good health.[33] This process, performed by a forensic pathologist or other pathologist with appropriate experience, involves a full examination of the deceased and procurement of an antecedent clinical history and family history

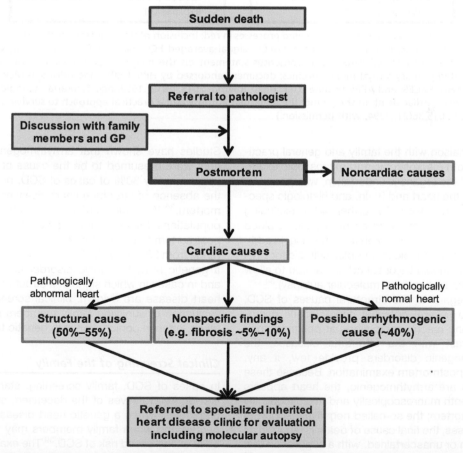

Fig. 1. The process following an SCD event (processes in red; potential findings in blue). GP, general practitioner.

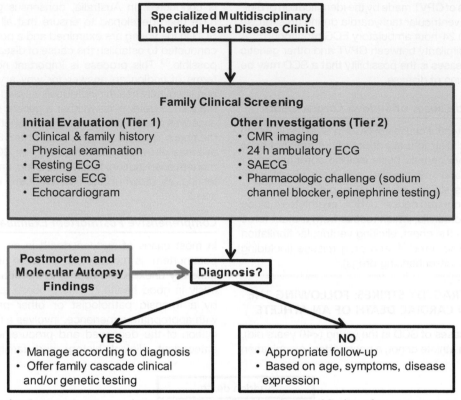

Fig. 2. The family screening process (screening processes in red; inclusion of findings from postmortem procedure in blue). CMR, cardiac magnetic resonance; SAECG, signal-averaged ECG. (*Adapted from* Priori SG, Wilde AA, Horie M, et al. HRS/EHRA/APHRS expert consensus statement on the diagnosis and management of patients with inherited primary arrhythmia syndromes: document endorsed by HRS, EHRA, and APHRS in May 2013 and by ACCF, AHA, PACES, and AEPC in June 2013. Heart Rhythm 2013;10(12):1952; and Semsarian C, Ingles J, Wilde AAM. Sudden cardiac death in the young: the molecular autopsy and a practical approach to surviving relatives. Eur Heart J 2015;36(21):1294; with permission.)

through liaison with the family and general practitioner. Both macroscopic and microscopic examination of the organs is undertaken, with particular focus on the heart and brain, and histologic specimens are reviewed. To further aid in excluding noncardiac causes, such as drug toxicity, blood and urine samples are taken for screening. In addition, tissue and/or blood samples suitable for DNA extraction should be obtained and stored to allow for genetic testing (ie, a molecular autopsy).[34]

With regard to the structural causes of SCD, there are several potential characteristic microscopic and macroscopic signs at postmortem.[35] In contrast with the structural diseases, the arrhythmogenic disorders provide few, if any, clues at postmortem examination. Because these diseases are arrhythmogenic, the heart appears normal both macroscopically and microscopically at postmortem; the so-called negative autopsy. In these cases, the final cause of death is reported as unknown or unascertained, with a suggestion that an arrhythmogenic disorder may be responsible.[36]

Studies have shown that arrhythmogenic disorders were presumed to be the cause of death in approximately 30% of cases of SCD, because of the absence of structural heart diseases at postmortem.[36,37] In studies of sudden death in athlete populations, the incidence of a negative finding at postmortem has been found to be similar, with a range from 23% to 31%.[5,23,31,38] In cases in which a genetic arrhythmogenic disorder is suspected and in cases in which signs of a structural genetic heart disease are evident, clinical screening and evaluation of surviving family members is undertaken, often in conjunction with genetic testing.

Clinical Screening of the Family

In cases of SCD, family screening, starting with first-degree relatives of the deceased, should be undertaken when a genetic heart disease is suspected and when family members may therefore be at an increased risk of SCD.[39] The exact nature of the clinical screening depends on the suspected disease; however, it should include clinical history, physical examination, ECG, echocardiogram, and in some cases an exercise stress test, as shown in **Fig. 2**.[34,39] In addition, a thorough family history should be compiled, taking particular note of any instances of unexplained syncope, seizures, and sudden deaths at a young age in family members.[34,39] Other investigations that may be considered include cardiac MRI, a 24-hour Holter monitor ECG, a signal-averaged ECG, and a pharmacologic challenge if Brugada syndrome is suspected.[34]

Role of the Molecular Autopsy

In addition to family screening, genetic testing can play a pivotal role in determining the cause of death, particularly in the approximately 30% of SCD cases that remain unascertained following postmortem. With arrhythmogenic disorders thought to be responsible for most of these deaths, postmortem genetic testing has the power to reveal disease-causing genes present in the deceased, or proband, providing not only the probable cause of death but also the opportunity for further genetic testing in living family members. Genetic testing in these cases involves extracting DNA from postmortem blood, analysis through Sanger sequencing, cardiac gene panels or whole-exome/genome sequencing, and identification of pathogenic (disease-causing) mutations.[34] Genetic testing using a panel of the major arrhythmogenic disease genes has been found to reveal disease-causing mutations in approximately 30% of cases of sudden unexplained death.[40] **Table 1** shows the major disease genes generally screened in the molecular autopsy for the genetic heart diseases.[40] Advances in next-generation genetic testing technologies have resulted in reducing costs, expediting delivery of test results, and the addition of new candidate genes to testing panels. Moreover, the development of an exome-wide molecular autopsy, in which the coding regions of all genes are sequenced, is allowing an even wider search for disease-causing genes, including those less commonly involved in disease.[40] In all cases in which a disease-causing gene mutation is identified in a proband, cascade genetic testing may be undertaken within the family to identify any individuals who carry the same gene and are at risk of having the same disease.

STILL MUCH TO LEARN

Although much is known about the causes of SCD, there is still much to learn. As mentioned, approximately one-third of SCD cases are unascertained

at postmortem. Of these, clinical and genetic screening may reveal a cause in 10% to 30% of cases,[40,41] leaving a substantial proportion unascertained despite thorough postmortem, genetic, and clinical examination. In these cases, family members are left with no answer for why their loved one died suddenly and are left to wonder whether the same thing will happen to them. It seems that despite the sizable advances made in the area of genetic testing and the use of the molecular autopsy, there is still much to learn; for example, in the discovery of new disease-causing gene mutations.

In addition to unknown cardiac pathogenic mutations, there are other causes that may not be identified in the current investigation process. For example, caffeine is often taken by athletes to enhance performance, whether in the form of coffee, tablets, or energy drinks.[42] However, caffeine can act within myocytes, inducing similar effects to that of adrenaline,[43] and cases have been reported in which individuals have experienced adverse cardiac events following ingestion of energy drinks.[44] Ma huang (a source of ephedrine), a herbal supplement, may also be taken by athletes for its perceived stimulant effect; however, it has also been implicated in cases of SCD.[45] Other pharmaceutical drugs may also be responsible for SCD events and may not be picked up on toxicology screening during postmortem, such as those that prolong the QT interval.[46] Furthermore, illegal doping has also been implicated in SCD cases, most notably with the use of anabolic steroids and hormones.[47–49] The precise arrhythmogenic potential of these substances is unclear; however, most of the illicit drugs identified by the World Anti-Doping Agency are thought to have an arrhythmogenic effect.[48] In addition, with improvements in detection of illicit drug use, more substances are being developed to circumvent the detection processes. Until these substances can be identified, the nature of their cardiovascular effects will also remain elusive.

Other non–drug-related causes might also play a role in SCD in athletes but remain indefinable at postmortem. Heat stroke may be caused by an increased environmental temperature or be induced by exertion (ie, exercise), and can lead to cardiac arrhythmias.[50] In addition, the physiologic responses to exercise, such as electrolyte imbalances, increased catecholamine levels, dehydration, and acidosis, may all act as triggers for potentially lethal arrhythmias.[16] In some cases, these causes may not be identified at postmortem and therefore the cause of death remains unknown.

At the level of the postmortem examination, studies have identified a further potential area for growth in knowledge. Although it may be perceived that a physical postmortem examination should provide a certain diagnosis in cases of SCD with an underlying structural disease, studies have shown that there is often uncertainty. In a study of collegiate-level athletes in the United States, a multidisciplinary panel, comprising individuals with extensive experience in SCD in athletes, examined 45 cases of SCD.[31] The study involved a thorough assessment of postmortem reports and the diagnosis of the expert panel concurred with that of the postmortem report in only 60% of cases. It was observed that the quality of the autopsies varied substantially and that the training and expertise of those conducting the autopsies varied by location. A study from Italy found that 79% of deaths, in which individuals were categorized as having pathologically normal hearts on macroscopic examination, were later found to have a specific cause following closer evaluation.[51] These studies suggest that the postmortem is fallible and is reliant on the experience and expertise of the pathologist conducting the examination. It may be that some cases that are deemed unascertained by an inexperienced pathologist might have a structural cause that would have been found by a pathologist with more expertise. In addition, alternate or supplementary techniques should be investigated. A recent study of 17 cases of SCD in young people compared the conventional postmortem procedure with MRI and computed tomography as a means of determining the cause of death.[52] The initial data from this and other studies[53] show the potential of imaging techniques in establishing the cause of SCD.

Related perhaps to the dependability of postmortem conclusions, across the world there have been differences observed between the incidences of various causes of SCD and also in the rates of diagnosis following postmortem. Harmon and colleagues[31] identified 6 studies of SCD in athletes and 2 studies of SCD in military populations, and observed a range in incidences of various causes. For example, the incidence of HCM ranged from 0% to 36% of individuals, the incidence of ARVC ranged from 1% to 27%, and the incidence of postmortem negative findings ranged from 7% to 41%. The reasons behind these considerable differences are unknown and thus there is still much to discover and learn with regard to this issue.

Perhaps the most stark and contentious difference is seen between studies from Italy and those from the United States, which provide the extremes of the ranges discussed earlier. A 21-year prospective study of all young people in the Veneto region of Italy found 55 sudden deaths in athletes, of which most (22%) were caused by ARVC.[13] However, a study of 1866 sudden deaths of young, competitive athletes in the United States found that most deaths were caused by HCM (36%), with only 4% attributed to ARVC.[5] As mentioned, the reasons for these differences are yet to be confirmed, with the Italian group proposing that a genetic factor, such as a higher prevalence of ARVC caused by the homogenous nature of the study population (ie, from a well-defined area), has led to a higher incidence of SCD caused by ARVC.[13] However, higher prevalence of ARVC in the population in the Veneto region has not been established. Alternatively, the hypothesis is put forward that, because of the difficulties in diagnosing ARVC at postmortem, several SCD cases with no apparent cause may have been caused by ARVC.[13] This hypothesis again highlights the importance of improving education and increasing awareness among less-experienced pathologists conducting postmortem examinations.

Although it is important to establish reliable and consistent processes and techniques to determine cause of death following an SCD, it would be even better to prevent SCD occurring. As mentioned earlier, many of the potential causes of SCD in athletes present with features on clinical evaluation. As such, some clinicians advocate preparticipation screening for competitive athletes in order to detect cardiovascular abnormalities and the athletes at risk of SCD before it happens.[54] However, intense exercise has the potential to lead to structural and electrical remodeling of the heart, such as cardiac enlargement and abnormal patterns on ECG.[55] The presence of this gray zone between the benign adaptions or athlete's heart and the pathogenic changes of the genetic heart diseases makes preparticipation screening difficult, particularly when an ECG is included as part of the process. Criteria have been developed in order to aid clinicians in distinguishing between benign and potentially pathogenic changes on ECG.[56,57] However, there is still more to learn, with several false-positives still occurring, meaning that athletes may be unnecessarily excluded from their chosen sports. In contrast, because the process is fallible, some athletes may be cleared to play only to tragically experience SCD later in their careers.

SUMMARY

SCD in young athletes, often perceived as the epitome of health and vitality, are tragic and confronting events for those involved. With an incidence of 1 to 3 per 100,000 athletes, these events are rare; however, given the potential flow-on effects for family members, it is vitally important that clinicians involved in SCD cases are well informed. If an individual is diagnosed with a genetic heart disease, family members have a 1 in 2 chance of also having the same disease. Therefore, it is imperative that these diseases are identified when present in SCD cases, either at postmortem, family clinical screening, or from genetic testing. However, even with advances in technologies such as genetic testing, the cause of SCD may remain unascertained despite thorough investigation. There is still much to learn about SCD in athletes, most particularly in the determination of cause of death at postmortem and through genetic testing.

REFERENCES

1. Semsarian C, Sweeting J, Ackerman MJ. Sudden cardiac death in athletes. BMJ 2015;350:h1218.
2. Maron BJ. Sudden death in young athletes. N Engl J Med 2003;349(11):1064–75.
3. Sweeting J, Ingles J, Ball K, et al. Sudden deaths during the largest community running event in Australia: a 25-year review. Int J Cardiol 2015;203:1029–31.
4. Adabag AS, Luepker RV, Roger VL, et al. Sudden cardiac death: epidemiology and risk factors. Nat Rev Cardiol 2010;7(4):216–25.
5. Maron BJ, Doerer JJ, Haas TS, et al. Sudden deaths in young competitive athletes: analysis of 1866 deaths in the United States, 1980-2006. Circulation 2009;119(8):1085–92.
6. Maron BJ, Zipes DP. Introduction: eligibility recommendations for competitive athletes with cardiovascular abnormalities-general considerations. J Am Coll Cardiol 2005;45(8):1318–21.
7. Solberg EE, Borjesson M, Sharma S, et al. Sudden cardiac arrest in sports - need for uniform registration: a position paper from the sport cardiology section of the European Association for Cardiovascular Prevention and Rehabilitation. Eur J Prev Cardiol 2016;23(6):657–67.
8. Harmon KG, Drezner JA, Wilson MG, et al. Incidence of sudden cardiac death in athletes: a state-of-the-art review. Br J Sports Med 2014;48(15):1185–92.
9. Harmon KG, Asif IM, Maleszewski JJ, et al. Incidence, cause, and comparative frequency of sudden cardiac death in National Collegiate Athletic Association Athletes. Circulation 2015;132(1):10–9.
10. Maron BJ, Haas TS, Murphy CJ, et al. Incidence and causes of sudden death in U.S. college athletes. J Am Coll Cardiol 2014;63(16):1636–43.
11. Holst AG, Winkel BG, Theilade J, et al. Incidence and etiology of sports-related sudden cardiac death in Denmark–implications for preparticipation screening. Heart Rhythm 2010;7(10):1365–71.
12. Risgaard B, Winkel BG, Jabbari R, et al. Sports-related sudden cardiac death in a competitive and a noncompetitive athlete population aged 12 to 49 years: data from an unselected nationwide study in Denmark. Heart Rhythm 2014;11(10):1673–81.
13. Corrado D, Basso C, Rizzoli G, et al. Does sports activity enhance the risk of sudden death in adolescents and young adults? J Am Coll Cardiol 2003;42(11):1959–63.
14. Harmon KG, Asif IM, Klossner D, et al. Incidence of sudden cardiac death in National Collegiate Athletic Association athletes. Circulation 2011;123(15):1594–600.
15. Corrado D, Migliore F, Basso C, et al. Exercise and the risk of sudden cardiac death. Herz 2006;31(6):553–8.
16. Heidbuchel H, Carre F. Exercise and competitive sports in patients with an implantable cardioverter-defibrillator. Eur Heart J 2014;35(44):3097–102.
17. Cirino AL, Ho CY. Genetic testing for inherited heart disease. Circulation 2013;128(1):e4–8.
18. Ackerman MJ, Zipes DP, Kovacs RJ, et al. Eligibility and disqualification recommendations for competitive athletes with cardiovascular abnormalities: Task Force 10: the cardiac channelopathies: a scientific statement from the American Heart Association and American College of Cardiology. Circulation 2015;132(22):e326–9.
19. Maron BJ, Udelson JE, Bonow RO, et al. Eligibility and disqualification recommendations for competitive athletes with cardiovascular abnormalities: Task Force 3: hypertrophic cardiomyopathy, arrhythmogenic right ventricular cardiomyopathy and other cardiomyopathies, and myocarditis: a scientific statement from the American Heart Association and American College of Cardiology. J Am Coll Cardiol 2015;66(21):2362–71.
20. Maron BJ. Hypertrophic cardiomyopathy: a systematic review. JAMA 2002;287(10):1308–20.
21. Maron BJ, Casey SA, Poliac LC, et al. Clinical course of hypertrophic cardiomyopathy in a regional United States cohort. JAMA 1999;281(7):650–5.
22. Semsarian C, Ingles J, Maron MS, et al. New perspectives on the prevalence of hypertrophic cardiomyopathy. J Am Coll Cardiol 2015;65(12):1249–54.
23. de Noronha SV, Sharma S, Papadakis M, et al. Aetiology of sudden cardiac death in athletes in the United Kingdom: a pathological study. Heart 2009;95(17):1409–14.
24. Drezner JA, Ashley E, Baggish AL, et al. Abnormal electrocardiographic findings in athletes: recognising changes suggestive of cardiomyopathy. Br J Sports Med 2013;47(3):137–52.

25. Calkins H. Arrhythmogenic right ventricular dysplasia. Curr Probl Cardiol 2013;38(3):103–23.

26. Schwartz PJ, Stramba-Badiale M, Crotti L, et al. Prevalence of the congenital long-QT syndrome. Circulation 2009;120(18):1761–7.

27. Liu N, Ruan Y, Priori SG. Catecholaminergic polymorphic ventricular tachycardia. Prog Cardiovasc Dis 2008;51(1):23–30.

28. Giudicessi JR, Ackerman MJ. Potassium-channel mutations and cardiac arrhythmias–diagnosis and therapy. Nat Rev Cardiol 2012;9(6):319–32.

29. Priori SG, Wilde AA, Horie M, et al. HRS/EHRA/APHRS expert consensus statement on the diagnosis and management of patients with inherited primary arrhythmia syndromes: document endorsed by HRS, EHRA, and APHRS in May 2013 and by ACCF, AHA, PACES, and AEPC in June 2013. Heart Rhythm 2013;10(12): 1932–63.

30. Darbar D. Triggers for cardiac events in patients with type 2 long QT syndrome. Heart Rhythm 2010;7(12): 1806–7.

31. Harmon KG, Drezner JA, Maleszewski JJ, et al. Pathogeneses of sudden cardiac death in National Collegiate Athletic Association athletes. Circ Arrhythm Electrophysiol 2014;7(2):198–204.

32. Maron BJ, Ahluwalia A, Haas TS, et al. Global epidemiology and demographics of commotio cordis. Heart Rhythm 2011;8(12):1969–71.

33. Royal College of Pathologists of Australasia. Post-mortem in sudden unexpected death in the young: guidelines on autopsy practice. 2008. Available at: https://http://www.rcpa.edu.au/getattachment/89884c69-f066-411d-a3d1-39460444db13/Guidelines-on-Autopsy-Practice.aspx. Accessed October 13, 2015.

34. Semsarian C, Ingles J, Wilde AAM. Sudden cardiac death in the young: the molecular autopsy and a practical approach to surviving relatives. Eur Heart J 2015;36(21):1290–6.

35. Corrado D, Basso C, Nava A, et al. Arrhythmogenic right ventricular cardiomyopathy: current diagnostic and management strategies. Cardiol Rev 2001;9(5): 259–65.

36. Doolan A, Langlois N, Semsarian C. Causes of sudden cardiac death in young Australians. Med J Aust 2004;180(3):110–2.

37. Winkel BG, Holst AG, Theilade J, et al. Nationwide study of sudden cardiac death in persons aged 1-35 years. Eur Heart J 2011;32(8):983–90.

38. Chappex N, Schlaepfer J, Fellmann F, et al. Sudden cardiac death among general population and sport related population in forensic experience. J Forensic Leg Med 2015;35:62–8.

39. Ingles J, Semsarian C. Sudden cardiac death in the young: a clinical genetic approach. Intern Med J 2007;37(1):32–7.

40. Bagnall RD, Das KJ, Duflou J, et al. Exome analysis-based molecular autopsy in cases of sudden unexplained death in the young. Heart Rhythm 2014; 11(4):655–62.

41. Tan HL, Hofman N, van Langen IM, et al. Sudden unexplained death: heritability and diagnostic yield of cardiological and genetic examination in surviving relatives. Circulation 2005;112(2):207–13.

42. Spriet LL. Exercise and sport performance with low doses of caffeine. Sports Med 2014;44(Suppl 2): S175–84.

43. Gunja N, Brown JA. Energy drinks: health risks and toxicity. Med J Aust 2012;196(1):46–9.

44. Gray B, Das KJ, Semsarian C. Consumption of energy drinks: a new provocation test for primary arrhythmogenic diseases? Int J Cardiol 2012;159(1): 77–8.

45. Samenuk D, Link MS, Homoud MK, et al. Adverse cardiovascular events temporally associated with ma huang, an herbal source of ephedrine. Mayo Clin Proc 2002;77(1):12–6.

46. Behr ER, Roden D. Drug-induced arrhythmia: pharmacogenomic prescribing? Eur Heart J 2013;34(2): 89–95.

47. Fineschi V, Riezzo I, Centini F, et al. Sudden cardiac death during anabolic steroid abuse: morphologic and toxicologic findings in two fatal cases of bodybuilders. Int J Legal Med 2007;121(1):48–53.

48. Furlanello F, Serdoz LV, Cappato R, et al. Illicit drugs and cardiac arrhythmias in athletes. Eur J Cardiovasc Prev Rehabil 2007;14(4):487–94.

49. Dhar R, Stout CW, Link MS, et al. Cardiovascular toxicities of performance-enhancing substances in sports. Mayo Clin Proc 2005;80(10):1307–15.

50. Bouchama A, Knochel JP. Heat stroke. N Engl J Med 2002;346(25):1978–88.

51. Corrado D, Basso C, Thiene G. Sudden cardiac death in young people with apparently normal heart. Cardiovasc Res 2001;50(2):399–408.

52. Puranik R, Gray B, Lackey H, et al. Comparison of conventional autopsy and magnetic resonance imaging in determining the cause of sudden death in the young. J Cardiovasc Magn Reson 2014;16:44.

53. Roberts IS, Benamore RE, Benbow EW, et al. Post-mortem imaging as an alternative to autopsy in the diagnosis of adult deaths: a validation study. Lancet 2012;379(9811):136–42.

54. Corrado D, Thiene G. Protagonist: routine screening of all athletes prior to participation in competitive sports should be mandatory to prevent sudden cardiac death. Heart Rhythm 2007;4(4):520–4.

55. Prior DL, La Gerche A. The athlete's heart. Heart 2012;98(12):947–55.

56. Corrado D, Pelliccia A, Heidbuchel H, et al. Recommendations for interpretation of 12-lead electrocardiogram in the athlete. Eur Heart J 2010;31(2): 243–59.

57. Drezner JA, Ackerman MJ, Anderson J, et al. Electrocardiographic interpretation in athletes: the 'Seattle Criteria'. Br J Sports Med 2013;47(3):122–4.

58. Wilde AA, Behr ER. Genetic testing for inherited cardiac disease. Nat Rev Cardiol 2013;10(10): 571–83.

59. Chandra N, Bastiaenen R, Papadakis M, et al. Sudden cardiac death in young athletes: practical challenges and diagnostic dilemmas. J Am Coll Cardiol 2013;61(10):1027–40.

60. Ehtisham J, Watkins H. Is Wolff-Parkinson-White syndrome a genetic disease? J Cardiovasc Electrophysiol 2005;16(11):1258–62.

61. Vohra J, Rajagopalan S. Update on the diagnosis and management of Brugada syndrome. Heart Lung Circ 2015;24(12):1141–8.

Using the 12-Lead Electrocardiogram in the Care of Athletic Patients

Tee Joo Yeo, MBBS, MRCP (UK)[a],
Sanjay Sharma, BSc, MD, FRCP (UK), FESC[b],*

KEYWORDS

- Sports cardiology • Preparticipation screening • Sudden cardiac death
- Electrocardiogram interpretation • Inherited cardiac disease

KEY POINTS

- The 12-lead electrocardiogram (ECG) in athletes differs significantly from that in nonathletes.
- Physiologic ECG abnormalities in athletes can overlap with potentially serious cardiac diseases, and efforts to differentiate between the two entities are continually being improved through contemporary ECG interpretation criteria.
- The benefits of detecting abnormalities and possibly preventing sudden cardiac death with ECG screening need to be balanced with variability in interpretation and the presence of cardiac diseases undetectable by ECG.

INTRODUCTION

More than 100 years after Einthoven's string galvanometer produced the first electrocardiogram (ECG) in a human, the 12-lead ECG (used interchangeably with ECG in this article) remains the cornerstone of diagnostic investigations in cardiology. Despite the advent of more technologically advanced imaging modalities, the ECG has maintained its status as an obligatory investigation in cardiology-related scenarios. The ECG's indispensable role is clearly shown in the care of athletes, in whom its use spans a myriad of possibilities from screening through to diagnosis, prognosis, risk stratification, and even possibly the prevention of sudden cardiac death (SCD).

DEFINITION OF AN ATHLETE

The American College of Cardiology and European Society of Cardiology (ESC) have similar qualitative definitions for a competitive athlete, namely a person who participates in regular competition, in which emphasis is placed on excellence and achievement, and systematic training is usually intense with a tendency for exertion to physical limits.[1,2] Although these definitions do not apply to noncompetitive, recreational, or leisure sports, the distinction between competitive and recreational athletes has been blurred with increasing participation rates and intensities of physical activity within the general population. Quantitative definitions have also been suggested in which an athlete is deemed to be a person who partakes in weekly intensive physical activity exceeding 4 to 10 hours.[3–5] The European Association for Cardiovascular Prevention and Rehabilitation acknowledges the need for inclusiveness by proposing that the definition of an athlete be based on the type, frequency, duration, and intensity of sport participation, as well as being categorized as competitive or recreational.[5]

Conflict of Interest: The authors have no conflict of interest or funding to disclose.
[a] Cardiac Department, National University Heart Centre, 1E Kent Ridge Road, Singapore 678267, Singapore;
[b] Cardiovascular & Cell Sciences Research Institute, St George's University of London, St George's University NHS Foundation Trust, Cranmer Terrace, London SW17 0RE, UK
* Corresponding author.
E-mail address: ssharma21@hotmail.com

Cardiol Clin 34 (2016) 543–555
http://dx.doi.org/10.1016/j.ccl.2016.06.004
0733-8651/16/© 2016 Elsevier Inc. All rights reserved.

ORIGINS OF THE ATHLETE'S HEART

As early as 1899, Henschen described cardiac enlargement in long distance skiers using basic percussion techniques, followed by Linzbach coining the term physiologic left ventricular hypertrophy (LVH) in 1947.[6] Since then, the constellation of physiologic, electrical, structural, and functional adaptations related to regular intensive physical activity have been termed the athlete's heart, and the ECG is ubiquitous in this definition. Electrocardiographic changes of rhythm disturbances and voltage criteria for ventricular hypertrophy were more frequently identified in athletes compared with the general population in small cohort studies between 1960 and 1990.[7] This trend continued into the twenty-first century as abnormal ECG patterns compatible with the presence of cardiovascular disease were observed in up to 40% of substantially large cohorts of athletes.[8] Expectedly, the spectrum of some ECG patterns in athletes includes overlap with those described in individuals with potentially serious cardiac diseases, thus creating a gray area in ECG interpretation. With such marked differences between the ECGs of athletes and those of non-athletes, the ability to differentiate physiology from disorder is critical, considering the young age of most athletes and the societal impact of SCD in sport.

THE ATHLETE'S ELECTROCARDIOGRAM

Bradyarrhythmias, such as sinus bradycardia greater than 30 beats/min (bpm), sinus arrhythmia, first-degree and second-degree (Mobitz type 1) atrioventricular block, wandering atrial pacemaker, and ectopic atrial rhythm, have been attributed to increased vagal tone following regular physical activity and are common in athletes (**Figs. 1** and **2**).[3] Increased vagal tone also manifests as ethnic-specific early repolarization changes. White athletes typically show concave ST segment elevation, whereas Afro-Caribbean/black athletes show convex ST segment elevation often associated with either biphasic or deep T-wave inversions (TWIs) in V1 to V4.[3] Isolated Sokolow-Lyon voltage criteria (combined amplitude of S wave in V1 [SV1] + largest R wave in V5 or 6 [RV5/6] ≥3.5 mV, or R wave in aVL ≥1.1 mV) for LVH and incomplete right bundle branch block (RBBB) are recognized manifestations of increased cardiac chamber size and wall thickness and regarded as normal physiologic adaptations in athletes.[3]

DETERMINANTS OF ELECTROCARDIOGRAM PATTERNS IN ATHLETES

The manifestations of athletes' ECGs are governed by several demographic factors, including sporting discipline (see **Fig. 2**).

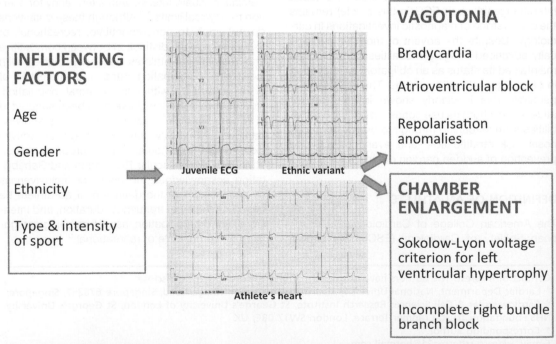

INFLUENCING FACTORS

Age

Gender

Ethnicity

Type & intensity of sport

Juvenile ECG   Ethnic variant   Athlete's heart

VAGOTONIA

Bradycardia

Atrioventricular block

Repolarisation anomalies

CHAMBER ENLARGEMENT

Sokolow-Lyon voltage criterion for left ventricular hypertrophy

Incomplete right bundle branch block

Fig. 1. Factors influencing athletes' ECGs and electrocardiographic manifestations of physiologic cardiac remodeling.

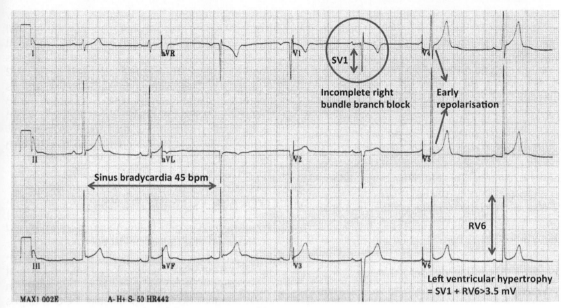

Fig. 2. Common training-related features in an athlete's ECG.

Age

The ECGs of adolescent/peripubertal athletes generally mirror those seen in postpubertal/adult athletes, with more frequent sinus bradycardia, low-grade atrioventricular block, partial RBBB, and voltage criteria for left and/or right ventricular hypertrophy than their nonathletic counterparts.[9]

Up to 8% of athletes less than 16 years old also manifest the juvenile ECG pattern; specifically, TWIs in V1 to V3 that are considered normal. These TWIs commonly revert to an upright morphology after puberty (**Fig. 3**).[10] However, TWIs are associated with cardiomyopathy in adults and may lead to diagnostic uncertainty in younger athletes with persistent TWI. In studies

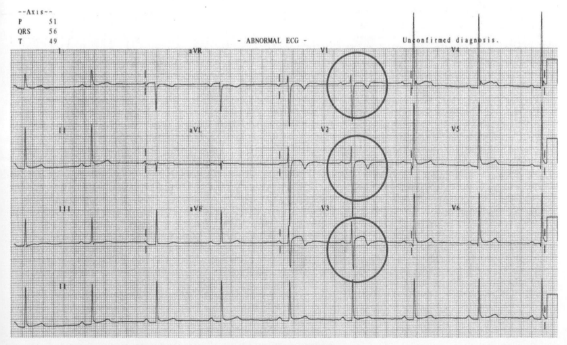

Fig. 3. An adolescent athlete's ECG showing juvenile TWI (*circled*).

examining large cohorts of peripubertal athletes, up to 2.5% of those with TWI, mostly in the inferolateral distribution, had significant structural abnormalities including potentially lethal cardiomyopathy.[10,11]

Gender

Abnormal ECG patterns are almost 4 times more likely in male athletes compared with their female counterparts. These patterns include higher prevalence rates of voltage criteria for LVH and repolarization changes.[8] This trend has been attributed to a decreased gender-related physiologic response to athletic training in female athletes.[12] In contrast, women have longer corrected QT (QTc) intervals than men and this holds true for the athletic population, leading to different gender-based cutoffs for normality.[3]

Ethnicity

Although early prevalence studies involved predominantly white athletes, the focus has shifted to black athletes with increasing emphasis on athletes from the Middle East and Asia.[13] Compared with athletes of other ethnicities, several aspects of the ECGs in black athletes often appear substantially abnormal, with more frequent repolarization abnormalities including TWI, voltage criteria for left and right ventricular hypertrophy, as well as left and right

atrial enlargement.[14] For instance, 1 in 8 healthy black athletes without cardiomyopathy show TWI in V1 to V4 associated with convex ST segment elevation, whereas only 0.2% of white athletes aged more than 16 years showed TWI beyond V2 (**Fig. 4**).[11,15] These differences show the enormous interethnic variation in physiologic adaptations to physical activity, the huge margin for error when extrapolating recommendations based on predominantly white cohorts, and the need to establish evidence-based ethnic-specific ECG norms.

TYPE AND INTENSITY OF SPORT

Athletes are a largely heterogeneous group based on the sport and training involved. Endurance athletes participating in sports with high dynamic demand are almost 9 times more likely to present with abnormal ECGs than those engaging in nonendurance sports.[8] Specifically, ECG changes such as right ventricular hypertrophy and deep TWI in V1 to V3 are more common in endurance athletes compared with nonendurance athletes and are attributed to physiologic right heart remodeling.[16] The amateur or elite status of an athlete and degree of athletic training also contribute to the athlete's ECG. Elite athletes typically show abnormal ECG changes more frequently than amateurs, whereas increased training leads to a higher

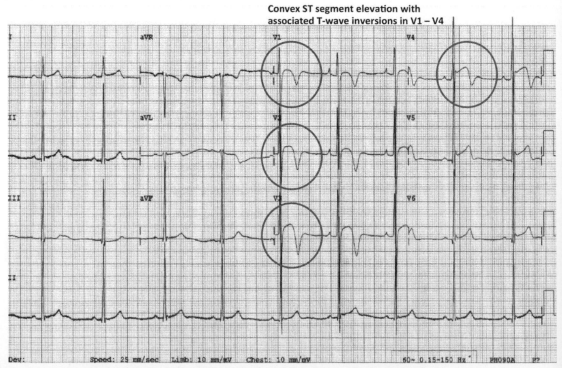

Convex ST segment elevation with associated T-wave inversions in V1 – V4

Fig. 4. A black athlete's ECG showing ethnic-specific repolarization changes (*circled*).

prevalence of ECG abnormalities such as early repolarization and RBBB.[17,18]

SUDDEN CARDIAC DEATH IN ATHLETES

Cardiovascular disease is the commonest cause of nontraumatic sudden death in sport. SCD affects approximately 1 in 50,000 athletes, with men and black athletes at highest risk.[19] Notably, population studies consistently report a higher risk of SCD in competitive athletes compared with their nonathletic counterparts or recreational sports participants, with relative risks up to 4.5.[20] Hypertrophic cardiomyopathy (HCM) has been established as the most frequent cause for sudden deaths in young athletes, accounting for 35% of deaths in the United States, whereas arrhythmogenic right ventricular cardiomyopathy (ARVC) has been implicated as the commonest cause in almost 30% of the deaths of young competitive athletes in the Veneto region of Italy.[21,22] Another major cause of SCD, accountable for 23% to 31% of athletes' deaths, is the sudden arrhythmic death syndrome, defined as an unexplained sudden death with normal cardiac pathology on autopsy and negative toxicology screen (**Fig. 5**).[23]

THE ELECTROCARDIOGRAM'S ROLE IN DIAGNOSIS, PROGNOSIS, AND RISK STRATIFICATION OF POTENTIALLY SERIOUS CARDIOVASCULAR ABNORMALITIES

The ECG identifies up to 63% of athletes who may be vulnerable to SCD.[24] This capability is vital given that up to 80% of SCDs in athletes have no antecedent symptoms or family history and the first clinical manifestation of an underlying cardiac disorder is sudden death.[23] Among athletes with HCM, more than 96% present with an abnormal ECG displaying distinctive features facilitating a diagnosis.[25] These features include TWI, pathologic Q waves, ST segment depression, left bundle branch block, left axis deviation, and left atrial enlargement (**Fig. 6**).[26] These features may precede the development of pathologic hypertrophy and allow an opportunity for early detection.[27] Up to 85% of individuals with ARVC show an abnormal ECG, with characteristic features including TWI in V1 to V3, epsilon waves, delayed S-wave upstroke, and low limb lead voltages (**Fig. 7**).[26] In a large Italian study, asymptomatic athletes expressing marked TWI on ECG but without apparent cardiac disease were followed up for 9 years and investigators detected cardiomyopathy (including HCM and ARVC) in 6%.[28] Apart from aiding diagnosis of potentially serious cardiovascular diseases, the ECG also plays a vital role in risk stratification. In patients with the long QT syndrome, a QTc greater than or equal to 500 milliseconds confers the highest risk of syncope, cardiac arrest, or sudden death.[29] In athletes with Brugada syndrome, a spontaneous type I pattern on ECG, defined as a coved-type ST segment elevation exceeding 2 mm, and QRS fragmentation seem to be associated with increased risk of syncope and sudden death.[30] For athletes with ventricular preexcitation, detection of paroxysmal atrioventricular reentry tachycardia, atrial fibrillation, or flutter may increase SCD risk, warranting catheter ablation before competitive sport participation.[31]

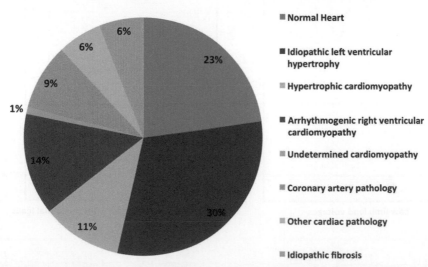

Fig. 5. Causes of SCD in athletes in the United Kingdom following pathologic assessment. (*From* de Noronha SV, Sharma S, Papadakis M, et al. Aetiology of sudden cardiac death in athletes in the United Kingdom: a pathological study. Heart 2009;95(17):1412; with permission.)

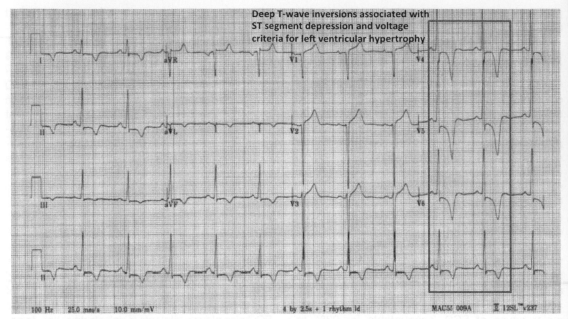

Fig. 6. ECG of an athlete with hypertrophic cardiomyopathy (characteristic features outlined within *red box*)..

THE EVOLUTION OF ELECTROCARDIOGRAM INTERPRETATION IN ATHLETES

The ability of the ECG to detect features suggestive of potentially serious cardiac diseases forms the basis of preparticipation screening of athletes in Europe and many other parts of the world (**Fig. 8**). Preparticipation screening with ECG is recommended by several major medical and sporting organizations, such as the ESC, International Olympic Committee, Federation Internationale de Football Association (FIFA), and various professional sporting leagues in the United

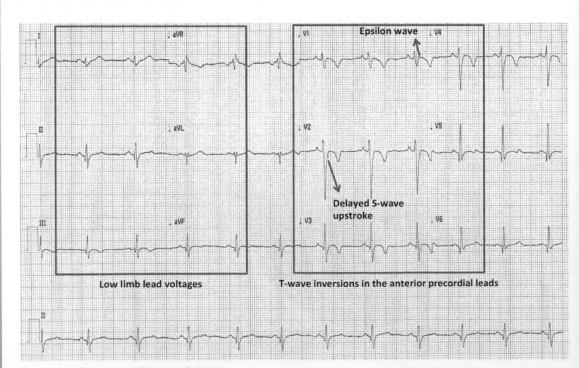

Fig. 7. ECG of a white athlete with ARVC.

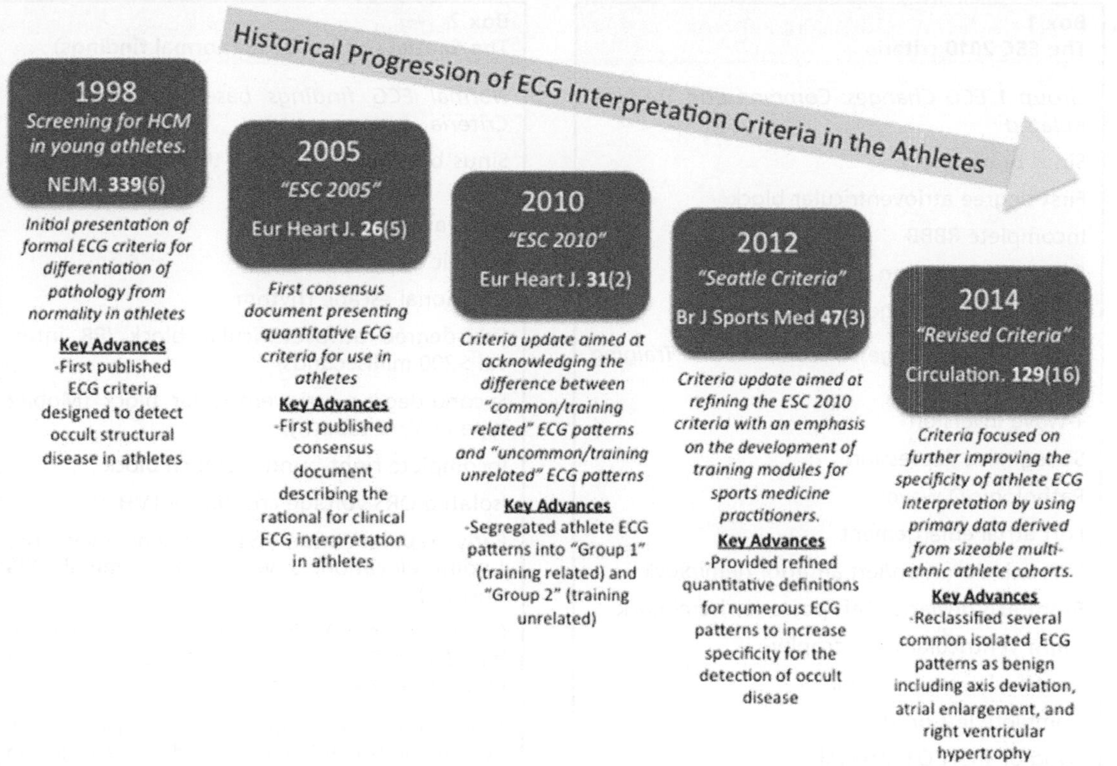

Fig. 8. The evolution of ECG interpretation in athletes. (*From* Baggish AL. A decade of athlete ECG criteria: where we've come and where we're going. J Electrocardiol 2015;48(3):325; with permission.)

States.[32] Detection of certain abnormal ECG features during athlete screening warrants further investigation to arrive at a confirmatory diagnosis. Recommendations pertaining to eligibility for continuation or disqualification from competitive sport depend on the severity of this diagnosis.[1,31]

THE EUROPEAN SOCIETY OF CARDIOLOGY CRITERIA

The earliest criteria for abnormal ECG findings in athletes was a compilation of previously described ECG features for a variety of cardiac disorders, including LVH and HCM (**Box 1**).[33] Notably, most of the criteria were dated and derived from abnormal findings in the general population rather than from athletes. Despite the capacity to detect all serious cardiac conditions requiring restriction of sporting activity, including a negative predictive value of 99.8% for HCM, false-positive rates were exceedingly high.[34]

Consequently, an improved document published in 2010 incorporated physiologic adaptations commonly encountered in athletes by classifying ECG abnormalities into common, training-related findings (Group 1) versus uncommon, training-unrelated changes (Group 2).[2] The 2010 criteria

improved specificity from 83% to 89.5% and reduced false-positives from 16.9% to 10% while preserving sensitivity.[35] Despite these improvements, significant ambiguity persisted and the number of false-positives remained unacceptably high, especially when applied to black athletes.

THE SEATTLE CRITERIA

In 2013, the Seattle Criteria provided quantitative cutoffs to aspects of athletes' ECGs not specified within the ESC document (**Box 2** and **Table 1**). Ethnicity-specific recommendations pertaining to TWI in black athletes were also incorporated based on prevalence studies in this population.[11,36–38] Thresholds for QTc intervals were amended, namely, the first ($\leq$320 milliseconds) and 99th ($\geq$470 milliseconds in men and $\geq$480 milliseconds in postpubertal women) percentiles of population norms were used as cutoffs for further evaluation of short and long QT syndromes respectively, leading to improved positive predictive values for ECG screening.[39] Abnormal ECG criteria were subdivided based on cardiac conditions responsible for SCD: the cardiomyopathies and primary electrical diseases. The criteria were structured to focus on helping sports physicians

Box 1
The ESC 2010 criteria

Group 1 ECG Changes: Common and Training Related

Sinus bradycardia

First-degree atrioventricular block

Incomplete RBBB

Early repolarization

Isolated QRS voltage criteria for LVH

Group 2 ECG Changes: Uncommon and Training Unrelated

T-wave inversion

ST segment depression

Pathologic Q waves

Left atrial enlargement

Left axis deviation/left anterior hemiblock

Right axis deviation/left posterior hemiblock

Right ventricular hypertrophy

Ventricular preexcitation

Complete left or RBBB

Long or short QT interval

Brugada-like early repolarization

From Corrado D, Pelliccia A, Heidbuchel H, et al. Recommendations for interpretation of 12-lead electrocardiogram in the athlete. Eur Heart J 2010;31:245; with permission.

Box 2
The Seattle Criteria 2013 (normal findings)

Normal ECG findings based on the Seattle Criteria

Sinus bradycardia greater than or equal to 30 bpm

Sinus arrhythmia

Ectopic atrial rhythm

Junctional escape rhythm

First-degree atrioventricular block (PR interval >200 milliseconds)

Second-degree atrioventricular block (Mobitz type I [Wenckebach])

Incomplete right bundle branch block

Isolated QRS voltage criteria for LVH

Early repolarization (ST segment elevation, J-point elevation, J waves, or terminal QRS slurring)

Convex (domed) ST segment elevation combined with T-wave inversion in leads V1 to V4 in black/African athletes

From Drezner JA, Fischbach P, Froelicher V, et al. Normal electrocardiographic findings: recognising physiological adaptations in athletes. Br J Sports Med 2013;47(3):126; with permission.

as well as cardiologists to differentiate normal from abnormal, and included an online training course for this purpose.[40] As a result of these revised contemporary limits for QTc intervals and TWI, the Seattle Criteria were consistently superior to the ESC criteria in specificity with further reduction in false-positives.[4,13,41,42]

THE REFINED CRITERIA

Continued progress in interpretation of athletes' ECGs brought attention to certain features, specifically left and right axis deviation, left and right atrial enlargement, and right ventricular hypertrophy (**Fig. 9**). These features were originally classified as abnormal based on evidence from the general, nonathletic population. As a unit, these features accounted for almost half of the ECG changes within group 2 of the ESC 2010 criteria but, when present in isolation, were not associated with any cardiac disorder in athlete-specific cohort studies.[43,44] Together with TWI preceded by convex ST segment elevation up to V4 in black

athletes, these 6 ECG patterns were classified as borderline, whereby no further evaluation was required if any of these were present in isolation, whereas the presence of 2 or more features warranted further investigation. These updated findings, combined with selected parameters from both ESC and Seattle Criteria, formed the basis of the Refined Criteria.[4] Application of the Refined Criteria has led to the largest reductions of false-positive rates to date, achieving 4.9% compared with 21.9% with the ESC criteria and 11.2% with the Seattle Criteria, in athletes of different ethnicities, while maintaining near-perfect sensitivity in detecting major cardiac abnormalities.[4,13]

FUTURE PROGRESS

To date, evidence comparing screening strategies favors the ECG as the most effective screening tool compared with history and physical examination.[45] With evolution of ECG interpretation in athletes, nuances in existing criteria continue to undergo scrutiny. Emerging evidence suggests that TWI beyond V4 combined with J-point elevation less than 1 mm independently predicts ARVC and HCM in black and white athletes.[46] The significance of anterior TWI in female athletes remains

Table 1
The Seattle Criteria 2013 (abnormal findings)

Abnormal ECG Finding	Definition
T-wave inversion	>1 mm in depth in 2 or more leads V2–V6, II and aVF, or I and aVL (excludes III, aVR, and V1)
ST segment depression	≥0.5 mm in depth in 2 or more leads
Pathologic Q waves	>3 mm in depth or >40 ms in duration in 2 or more leads (except for III and aVR)
Complete left bundle branch block	QRS ≥120 ms, predominantly negative QRS complex in lead V1 (QS or rS), and upright monophasic R wave in leads I and V6
Intraventricular conduction delay	Any QRS duration ≥140 ms
Left axis deviation	−30° to −90°
Left atrial enlargement	Prolonged P wave duration of >120 ms in leads I or II with negative portion of the P wave ≥1 mm in depth and ≥40 ms in duration in lead V1
Right ventricular hypertrophy pattern	R−V1+S−V5>10.5 mm and right axis deviation >120°
Ventricular preexcitation	PR interval <120 ms with a delta wave (slurred upstroke in the QRS complex) and wide QRS (>120 ms)
Long QT interval	QTc ≥470 ms (male) QTc ≥480 ms (female) QTc ≥500 ms (marked QT prolongation)
Short QT interval	QTc ≤320 ms
Brugada-like ECG pattern	High take-off and downsloping ST segment elevation followed by a negative T wave in ≥2 leads in V1–V3
Profound sinus bradycardia	<30 bpm or sinus pauses ≥3 s
Atrial tachyarrhythmias	Supraventricular tachycardia, atrial fibrillation, atrial flutter
Premature ventricular contractions	≥2 premature ventricular contractions per 10-s tracing
Ventricular arrhythmias	Couplets, triplets, and nonsustained ventricular tachycardia

From Drezner JA, Ackerman MJ, Anderson J, et al. Electrocardiographic interpretation in athletes: the 'Seattle Criteria'. Br J Sports Med 2013;47(3):123; with permission.

unclear given evolving data showing higher prevalence of TWI beyond V2 in female compared with male athletes.[47] In addition, the impact of differing cutoffs for QRS duration and degree of ST segment depression are also being studied and will contribute to information already available in the quest for ideal ECG interpretation criteria.[48]

DOES ELECTROCARDIOGRAM SCREENING SAVE LIVES?

Compelling evidence supporting ECG-based preparticipation screening in athletes comes from the Veneto region of Italy.[49] Researchers studied trends of SCD over 26 years in athletes aged 12 to 35 years before and after implementing a mandatory ECG-based athlete screening program. Rates of SCD in athletes decreased by 90% from 3.6 per 100,000 person-years before initiation of the screening program in 1979 to 1980 compared with 0.4 per 100000 person-

years in 2003 to 2004, by which time the program was well established. This improvement was attributed to identification of athletes with potentially lethal cardiac diseases and their ensuing disqualification from competitive activity. Comparatively, the rate of SCD in nonathletes in the same age group remained stable throughout the study period at 0.79 per 100,000 person-years, further supporting the efficacy of athlete screening.

In contrast, researchers in Israel reported that mandatory ECG screening of athletes did not reduce risk of SCD based on local data spanning more than 2 decades.[50] SCD rates for athletes averaged 2.54 per 100,000 years in the 10 years before legislation was passed in 1997 mandating ECG screening for athletes, whereas the incidence remained similar in the 10 years after legislation at 2.66 per 100,000 years, showing no apparent benefit of screening. A key difference between the two studies was that, in Italy, cases of SCD received an autopsy-based diagnosis and were

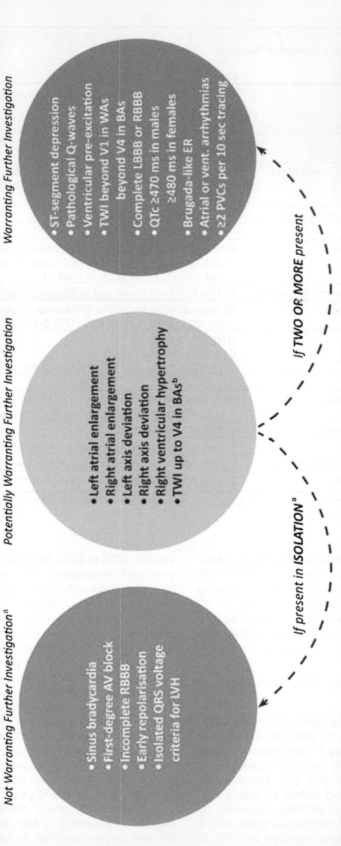

Refined Criteria Training Related Normal Variants
Not Warranting Further Investigation[a]

- Sinus bradycardia
- First-degree AV block
- Incomplete RBBB
- Early repolarisation
- Isolated QRS voltage criteria for LVH

If present in ISOLATION[a]

Refined Criteria Borderline Variants
Potentially Warranting Further Investigation

- Left atrial enlargement
- Right atrial enlargement
- Left axis deviation
- Right axis deviation
- Right ventricular hypertrophy
- TWI up to V4 in BAs[b]

If TWO OR MORE present

Refined Criteria Training Unrelated Changes
Warranting Further Investigation

- ST-segment depression
- Pathological Q-waves
- Ventricular pre-excitation
- TWI beyond V1 in WAs beyond V4 in BAs
- Complete LBBB or RBBB
- QTc ≥470 ms in males ≥480 ms in females
- Brugada-like ER
- Atrial or vent. arrhythmias
- ≥2 PVCs per 10 sec tracing

Fig. 9. The refined criteria 2014. AV, atrioventricular; BAs, black athletes; ER, early repolarisation; RBBB, right bundle branch block; TWI, T-wave inversion; WAs, white athletes. [a] in otherwise asymptomatic athletes with no family history or abnormal examination findings. [b] when preceded by characteristic convex ST-segment elevation. (*From* Sheikh N, Papadakis M, Ghani S, et al. Comparison of electrocardiographic criteria for the detection of cardiac abnormalities in elite black and white athletes. Circulation 2014;129(16):1638; with permission.)

tabulated from a national registry, whereas in Israel scrutinizing of media reports from 2 newspapers was the method used to search for SCD in athletes.

LIMITATIONS OF THE ELECTROCARDIOGRAM
Variation in Interpretation

The weakness of the athletes' ECG is the potential for wide variations in interpretation between readers. Studies assessing variability in interpretation of athletes' ECGs between doctors of varying specialties consistently reveal poor to moderate agreement at best, even after instructions for various ECG screening criteria were provided.[51,52] These findings stem from failure to agree on abnormality (agreement rates 38%–65%) and reflect the difficulty in ECG interpretation, even among trained specialists. Methods to improve these dismal values have been attempted with varying degrees of success, including interpretation tools and computer-based measurements.[53,54]

Cardiac Conditions Undetectable by Electrocardiogram

There remains a significant proportion of conditions capable of causing SCD in athletes that cannot be detected by ECG, specifically congenital and acquired coronary diseases such as coronary artery anomalies, the aortopathies and some ion channel diseases, including catecholaminergic polymorphic ventricular tachycardia.

MASTERS ATHLETES

In masters athletes, typically defined as greater than or equal to 35 years old, the incidence of SCD has been reported as significantly higher than in their younger counterparts, ranging between 1:15,000 and 1:50,000 per year.[55] Almost all SCD in masters athletes is caused by atherosclerotic coronary artery disease following the accumulation of traditional cardiovascular risk factors with age.[56] Up to 56% of those greater than or equal to 35 years old with sudden cardiac arrest during sports activity were found to have 1 or more risk factors for atherosclerosis.[57] The ECG has poor sensitivity and specificity to detect coronary artery disease and myocardial ischemia, and thus has limited utility. Nonetheless, ECG features identified as abnormal/training unrelated in younger athletes can be similarly applied to masters athletes to aid recognition of inherited cardiomyopathies and electrical disease despite lower incidence rates.[55] The utility of ECG screening for screening middle-aged athletes has not been formally tested but its role in evaluating athletes

with symptoms is likely to be as important as in younger athletes.

SUMMARY

The ECG, one of the oldest investigations in cardiology, continues to stay relevant in the care of athletes. Although it has proved to be a valuable resource in differentiating physiologic changes as a result of physical training from cardiac disorders, further diminishing the gray area between normal and abnormal remains a constant challenge. SCD in athletes is a genuine concern and future emphasis is imperative on contemporary cohorts in which data are currently less robust, such as adolescents, women, Asians, and athletes of mixed ethnicity. Enhancement of existing ECG interpretation criteria with potential reduction in variability in interpretation and false-positives may positively affect the ongoing debate on mandatory ECG screening for the athletic population.

REFERENCES

1. Maron BJ, Zipes DP, Kovacs RJ. Eligibility and disqualification recommendations for competitive athletes with cardiovascular abnormalities: preamble, principles, and general considerations: a scientific statement from the American Heart Association and American College of Cardiology. J Am Coll Cardiol 2015;66(21):2343–9.
2. Corrado D, Pelliccia A, Heidbuchel H, et al. Recommendations for interpretation of 12-lead electrocardiogram in the athlete. Eur Heart J 2010;31(2):243–59.
3. Drezner JA, Fischbach P, Froelicher V, et al. Normal electrocardiographic findings: recognising physiological adaptations in athletes. Br J Sports Med 2013;47(3):125–36.
4. Sheikh N, Papadakis M, Ghani S, et al. Comparison of electrocardiographic criteria for the detection of cardiac abnormalities in elite black and white athletes. Circulation 2014;129(16):1637–49.
5. Solberg EE, Borjesson M, Sharma S, et al. Sudden cardiac arrest in sports - need for uniform registration: a position paper from the sport cardiology section of the European Association for Cardiovascular Prevention and Rehabilitation. Eur J Prev Cardiol 2016;23(6):657–67.
6. Rost R. The athlete's heart. Eur Heart J 1982;3(Suppl A):193–8.
7. Huston TP, Puffer JC, Rodney WM. The athletic heart syndrome. N Engl J Med 1985;313(1):24–32.
8. Pelliccia A, Maron BJ, Culasso F, et al. Clinical significance of abnormal electrocardiographic patterns in trained athletes. Circulation 2000;102(3):278–84.

9. Sharma S, Whyte G, Elliott P, et al. Electrocardiographic changes in 1000 highly trained junior elite athletes. Br J Sports Med 1999;33(5):319–24.

10. Migliore F, Zorzi A, Michieli P, et al. Prevalence of cardiomyopathy in Italian asymptomatic children with electrocardiographic T-wave inversion at preparticipation screening. Circulation 2012;125(3):529–38.

11. Papadakis M, Basavarajaiah S, Rawlins J, et al. Prevalence and significance of T-wave inversions in predominantly Caucasian adolescent athletes. Eur Heart J 2009;30(14):1728–35.

12. Pelliccia A, Maron BJ, Culasso F, et al. Athlete's heart in women. Echocardiographic characterization of highly trained elite female athletes. JAMA 1996; 276(3):211–5.

13. Riding NR, Sheikh N, Adamuz C, et al. Comparison of three current sets of electrocardiographic interpretation criteria for use in screening athletes. Heart 2015;101(5):384–90.

14. Sheikh N, Sharma S. Impact of ethnicity on cardiac adaptation to exercise. Nat Rev Cardiol 2014;11(4): 198–217.

15. Papadakis M, Carre F, Kervio G, et al. The prevalence, distribution, and clinical outcomes of electrocardiographic repolarization patterns in male athletes of African/Afro-Caribbean origin. Eur Heart J 2011; 32(18):2304–13.

16. Brosnan M, La Gerche A, Kalman J, et al. Comparison of frequency of significant electrocardiographic abnormalities in endurance versus nonendurance athletes. Am J Cardiol 2014;113(9):1567–73.

17. Noseworthy PA, Weiner R, Kim J, et al. Early repolarization pattern in competitive athletes: clinical correlates and the effects of exercise training. Circ Arrhythm Electrophysiol 2011;4(4):432–40.

18. Kim JH, Noseworthy PA, McCarty D, et al. Significance of electrocardiographic right bundle branch block in trained athletes. Am J Cardiol 2011; 107(7):1083–9.

19. Harmon KG, Drezner JA, Wilson MG, et al. Incidence of sudden cardiac death in athletes: a state-of-the-art review. Br J Sports Med 2014; 48(15):1185–92.

20. Marijon E, Tafflet M, Celermajer DS, et al. Sports-related sudden death in the general population. Circulation 2011;124(6):672–81.

21. Maron BJ, Doerer JJ, Haas TS, et al. Sudden deaths in young competitive athletes: analysis of 1866 deaths in the United States, 1980-2006. Circulation 2009;119(8):1085–92.

22. Corrado D, Thiene G, Nava A, et al. Sudden death in young competitive athletes: clinicopathologic correlations in 22 cases. Am J Med 1990;89(5):588–96.

23. de Noronha SV, Sharma S, Papadakis M, et al. Aetiology of sudden cardiac death in athletes in the United Kingdom: a pathological study. Heart 2009; 95(17):1409–14.

24. Perez M, Fonda H, Le VV, et al. Adding an electrocardiogram to the pre-participation examination in competitive athletes: a systematic review. Curr Probl Cardiol 2009;34(12):586–662.

25. Sheikh N, Papadakis M, Schnell F, et al. Clinical profile of athletes with hypertrophic cardiomyopathy. Circ Cardiovasc Imaging 2015;8(7):e003454.

26. Drezner JA, Ashley E, Baggish AL, et al. Abnormal electrocardiographic findings in athletes: recognising changes suggestive of cardiomyopathy. Br J Sports Med 2013;47(3):137–52.

27. Gregor P, Widimsky P, Cervenka V, et al. Electrocardiographic changes can precede the development of myocardial hypertrophy in the setting of hypertrophic cardiomyopathy. Int J Cardiol 1989;23(3):335–41.

28. Pelliccia A, Di Paolo FM, Quattrini FM, et al. Outcomes in athletes with marked ECG repolarization abnormalities. N Engl J Med 2008;358(2):152–61.

29. Priori SG, Schwartz PJ, Napolitano C, et al. Risk stratification in the long-QT syndrome. N Engl J Med 2003;348(19):1866–74.

30. Delise P, Allocca G, Marras E, et al. Risk stratification in individuals with the Brugada type 1 ECG pattern without previous cardiac arrest: usefulness of a combined clinical and electrophysiologic approach. Eur Heart J 2011;32(2):169–76.

31. Pelliccia A, Fagard R, Bjornstad HH, et al. Recommendations for competitive sports participation in athletes with cardiovascular disease: a consensus document from the Study Group of Sports Cardiology of the Working Group of Cardiac Rehabilitation and Exercise Physiology and the Working Group of Myocardial and Pericardial Diseases of the European Society of Cardiology. Eur Heart J 2005;26(14):1422–45.

32. Bille K, Figueiras D, Schamasch P, et al. Sudden cardiac death in athletes: the Lausanne Recommendations. Eur J Cardiovasc Prev Rehabil 2006;13(6): 859–75.

33. Corrado D, Basso C, Schiavon M, et al. Screening for hypertrophic cardiomyopathy in young athletes. N Engl J Med 1998;339(6):364–9.

34. Baggish AL, Hutter AM Jr, Wang F, et al. Cardiovascular screening in college athletes with and without electrocardiography: a cross-sectional study. Ann Intern Med 2010;152(5):269–75.

35. Weiner RB, Hutter AM, Wang F, et al. Performance of the 2010 European Society of Cardiology criteria for ECG interpretation in athletes. Heart 2011;97(19): 1573–7.

36. Rawlins J, Carre F, Kervio G, et al. Ethnic differences in physiological cardiac adaptation to intense physical exercise in highly trained female athletes. Circulation 2010;121(9):1078–85.

37. Di Paolo FM, Schmied C, Zerguini YA, et al. The athlete's heart in adolescent Africans: an electrocardiographic and echocardiographic study. J Am Coll Cardiol 2012;59(11):1029–36.

38. Sheikh N, Papadakis M, Carre F, et al. Cardiac adaptation to exercise in adolescent athletes of African ethnicity: an emergent elite athletic population. Br J Sports Med 2013;47(9):585–92.

39. Drezner JA, Ackerman MJ, Cannon BC, et al. Abnormal electrocardiographic findings in athletes: recognising changes suggestive of primary electrical disease. Br J Sports Med 2013;47(3):153–67.

40. Drezner JA, Ackerman MJ, Anderson J, et al. Electrocardiographic interpretation in athletes: the 'Seattle Criteria'. Br J Sports Med 2013;47(3):122–4.

41. Wasfy MM, DeLuca J, Wang F, et al. ECG findings in competitive rowers: normative data and the prevalence of abnormalities using contemporary screening recommendations. Br J Sports Med 2015;49(3):200–6.

42. Brosnan M, La Gerche A, Kalman J, et al. The Seattle Criteria increase the specificity of preparticipation ECG screening among elite athletes. Br J Sports Med 2014;48(15):1144–50.

43. Gati S, Sheikh N, Ghani S, et al. Should axis deviation or atrial enlargement be categorised as abnormal in young athletes? The athlete's electrocardiogram: time for re-appraisal of markers of pathology. Eur Heart J 2013;34(47):3641–8.

44. Zaidi A, Ghani S, Sheikh N, et al. Clinical significance of electrocardiographic right ventricular hypertrophy in athletes: comparison with arrhythmogenic right ventricular cardiomyopathy and pulmonary hypertension. Eur Heart J 2013;34(47):3649–56.

45. Harmon KG, Zigman M, Drezner JA. The effectiveness of screening history, physical exam, and ECG to detect potentially lethal cardiac disorders in athletes: a systematic review/meta-analysis. J Electrocardiol 2015;48(3):329–38.

46. Calore C, Zorzi A, Sheikh N, et al. Electrocardiographic anterior T-wave inversion in athletes of different ethnicities: differential diagnosis between athlete's heart and cardiomyopathy. Eur Heart J 2015. [Epub ahead of print].

47. Malhotra A, Dhutia H, Gati S, et al. 103 prevalence and significance of anterior T wave inversion in females. Heart 2014;100(Suppl 3):A60.

48. Dunn T, Abdelfattah R, Aggarwal S, et al. Are the QRS duration and ST depression cut-points from the Seattle Criteria too conservative? J Electrocardiol 2015;48(3):395–8.

49. Corrado D, Basso C, Pavei A, et al. Trends in sudden cardiovascular death in young competitive athletes after implementation of a preparticipation screening program. JAMA 2006;296(13):1593–601.

50. Steinvil A, Chundadze T, Zeltser D, et al. Mandatory electrocardiographic screening of athletes to reduce their risk for sudden death proven fact or wishful thinking? J Am Coll Cardiol 2011;57(11):1291–6.

51. Berte B, Duytschaever M, Elices J, et al. Variability in interpretation of the electrocardiogram in young athletes: an unrecognized obstacle for electrocardiogram-based screening protocols. Europace 2015;17(9):1435–40.

52. Brosnan M, La Gerche A, Kumar S, et al. Modest agreement in ECG interpretation limits the application of ECG screening in young athletes. Heart Rhythm 2015;12(1):130–6.

53. Exeter DJ, Elley CR, Fulcher ML, et al. Standardised criteria improve accuracy of ECG interpretation in competitive athletes: a randomised controlled trial. Br J Sports Med 2014;48(15):1167–71.

54. Berge HM, Steine K, Andersen TE, et al. Visual or computer-based measurements: important for interpretation of athletes' ECG. Br J Sports Med 2014;48(9):761–7.

55. Maron BJ, Araujo CG, Thompson PD, et al. Recommendations for preparticipation screening and the assessment of cardiovascular disease in masters athletes: an advisory for healthcare professionals from the working groups of the World Heart Federation, the International Federation of Sports Medicine, and the American Heart Association Committee on Exercise, Cardiac Rehabilitation, and Prevention. Circulation 2001;103(2):327–34.

56. Whiteson JH, Bartels MN, Kim H, et al. Coronary artery disease in masters-level athletes. Arch Phys Med Rehabil 2006;87(3 Suppl 1):S79–81 [quiz: S2–3].

57. Marijon E, Uy-Evanado A, Reinier K, et al. Sudden cardiac arrest during sports activity in middle age. Circulation 2015;131(16):1384–91.

Exercise-Induced Atrial Remodeling
The Forgotten Chamber

Antonello D'Andrea, MD, PhD[a,*], Eduardo Bossone, MD[b],
Juri Radmilovic, MD[a], Lucia Riegler, MD[a],
Enrica Pezzullo, MD[a], Raffaella Scarafile, MD[a],
Maria Giovanna Russo, MD[a], Maurizio Galderisi, MD[c],
Raffaele Calabrò, MD[a]

KEYWORDS

- Athlete's heart • Left atrium • Left atrial volume • Speckle tracking • Diastole • Endurance
- Atrial fibrillation • Sport training

KEY POINTS

- The left atrium is not a symmetrically shaped 3-dimensional structure, so true left atrial size in athletes is more accurately reflected by a measurement of volume rather than area or linear dimension.
- In large populations of highly trained athletes, mild left atrial enlargement found by echocardiography (ECG) is relatively common (20% of patients) and may be identified as a physiologic adaptation to exercise conditioning.
- In both young and adult athletes, atrial abnormalities by ECG should be regarded as abnormal and lead to secondary investigation.
- Left atrial myocardial deformation assessed by strain is normal in elite athletes compared with age-matched sedentary controls and hypertensive patients, and is closely associated with functional capacity.
- Left atrial remodeling is associated with a higher risk of atrial fibrillation, especially in middle-aged male athletes with a history of intensive long-term endurance training.

BACKGROUND

The left atrium (LA) is located in the mediastinum, oriented leftward and posterior to the right atrium (RA). Its structure is characterized by a pulmonary venous component, a lateral appendage, an inferior vestibular component, and a prominent body that shares the septum with the RA.[1]

Clinical and echocardiographic evaluation of the LA can be essential for understanding many cardiac and noncardiac diseases. In fact, early detection of LA dysfunction provides new insight into pathophysiology and clinical management of several conditions such as atrial fibrillation (AF), arterial hypertension, heart failure, valvular heart disease, and cardiomyopathies.[1,2]

The athlete's heart is a cardiac adaptation to long-term exercise, characterized by an increase in wall thickness, cavity diameters, and left ventricular (LV) mass.[3–5]

Cardiac changes consist of morphologic and functional modifications, involving not only the left ventricle but also the LA. An increase of LA

[a] Department of Cardiology, Monaldi Hospital, Second University of Naples, Naples, Italy; [b] Department of Cardiology and Cardiac Surgery, University Hospital San Giovanni di Dio e Ruggi d'Aragona, Salern, Italy; [c] Department of Advanced Biomedical Sciences, Federico II University Hospital, Naples, Italy
* Corresponding author. Corso Vittorio Emanuele 121A, Naples 80121, Italy.
E-mail address: antonellodandrea@libero.it

Cardiol Clin 34 (2016) 557–565
http://dx.doi.org/10.1016/j.ccl.2016.06.005
0733-8651/16/© 2016 Elsevier Inc. All rights reserved.

dimensions in trained athletes may represent another component of the athlete's heart and upper limits should be used to distinguish physiologic and pathologic cardiac remodeling.[3–5]

LA enlargement is a predictor of AF in the general population and in patients with structural cardiac disease. The prevalence of LA remodeling and the association with supraventricular arrhythmias has not been systematically addressed in highly trained athletes.[6]

Echocardiography (ECG) is most frequently an appropriate second-level imaging modality for investigation of symptoms or screening abnormalities in the athlete. It can be helpful in distinguishing patients with disease involving LA morphology and function from those with LA remodeling concerning athlete's heart.[7] In addition, new echocardiographic techniques, such as Doppler myocardial imaging (DMI), speckle tracking, and 3-dimensional ECG are able to assess LA myocardial function and to identify early LA impairment in patients with either physiologic or pathologic LV hypertrophy (LVH).[5]

ECHOCARDIOGRAPHY ATRIAL ABNORMALITIES IN ATHLETES

Although by standard ECG the criterion for right atrial abnormality (RAA) is simple (P-wave amplitude >2.5 mm in II, II, or AVF leads), the criteria consistent with LA abnormality (LAA) are 2-fold: prolonged P-wave duration of greater than 120 ms in leads I or II with negative portion of the P wave greater than or equal to 1 mm in depth and greater than or equal to 40 ms in duration in lead V1.

Debate exists on the exact prevalence of atrial abnormality in athletes but it may be more common in younger athletes.[8–12] A prevalence of 14% and 18% for LAA and RAA, respectively, has been described in junior elite athletes.[8] This high prevalence is an anomaly within the literature and is unlikely to be explained by the age difference of the cohort alone. For example, in a similarly aged cohort of more than 1300 elite (national or international level) athletes, Brosnan and colleagues[11] observed a prevalence of LAA in 1.2% and 0.5% of endurance and nonendurance athletes, respectively, and the prevalence of RAA abnormalities was similar (1.2% and 0.3%, respectively). In other large cohorts, similarly low frequencies of abnormalities have been detected. In another population of 649 collegiate athletes with mean age of 20 years, LAA was seen in 0.7% and RAA in 1.8% of athletes.[10] Finally, Pelliccia and colleagues[9] found the prevalence of LAA to be 4% and RAA to be 0.8% in 1005 trained athletes.

As a consequence, in adult athletes, atrial abnormalities should be regarded as abnormal and lead to deeper investigation. Isolated atrial abnormalities in younger athletes should lead to a careful physical examination by a qualified physician, and to detailed personal medical and family history. Computerized measurements of total P-wave duration are not standardized, and visual assessment is still recommended.[12]

LEFT ATRIAL ECHOCARDIOGRAPHIC EVALUATION: FROM STANDARD MEASUREMENTS TO NEW ECHO TECHNOLOGIES

By standard ECG, the LA size can be traditionally measured at the end of ventricular systole, when the LA chamber has its greater dimension, in long axis view (anterior-posterior diameter), and in 4-chamber view (longitudinal and transverse diameters).[7]

However, linear measurements are considered to be inaccurate and do not represent true LA size because LA is not a symmetrically shaped 3-dimensional structure, so measurement of volume rather than area or linear dimension is preferred[2,7] (Fig. 1).

LA passive volumes consist of preatrial contraction volume (Vp), measured at the onset of the P-wave on an ECG; minimal LA volume (Vmin), measured at the closure of the mitral valve in end-diastole; and maximal LA volume (Vmax), measured just before the opening of the mitral valve in end-systole. LA active volumes are LA reservoir volume or LA filling volume (Vmax − Vmin); LA conduit volume or LA passive emptying volume (Vmax − Vp); and LA contractile volume (Vp − Vmin). The difference between maximum and minimum LA volume divided by the minimum LA volume is used as index of atrial compliance.[1]

Measurement of LA volume is recommended by ellipsoid model and Simpson method in 4-chamber and 2-chamber apical views. Normal indexed LA volume values for healthy sedentary subjects have been calculated in large population studies[7] (Fig. 2).

Mitral inflow patterns by pulsed wave Doppler examination demonstrate passive ventricular filling in early diastole (E velocity) and late active filling phase during atrial contraction (A velocity). Estimation of the peak A wave velocity is commonly used in studies that have evaluated atrial function.[13–15] By use of the standard Doppler analysis, one of the peculiar characteristics of the athlete's heart is that the increase of the LV mass verifies the absolute normality of

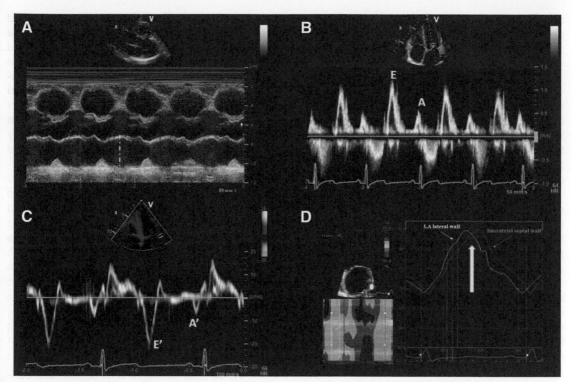

Fig. 1. LA morphologic and functional measurements: LA diameter (*A*), transmitral flow Doppler (*B*), Doppler tissue imaging (*C*), and strain curves (*D*).

both systolic and diastolic LV functional indexes. In particular, the transmitral inflow pattern of the athlete's heart demonstrates a supernormal aspect, with an increased volume of LV ventricular refill, which increases the contribution of early-diastolic phase in baseline conditions (E/A ratio >2). This feature helps to distinguish

pathologic and physiologic hypertrophy because in the former there is usually an impaired diastolic function (ie, E/A ratio <1, prolonged deceleration time)[16] (see **Fig. 1**).

By pulsed Doppler pulmonary venous flow can be recorded. The sample volume is placed into pulmonary veins (commonly right upper vein) by the

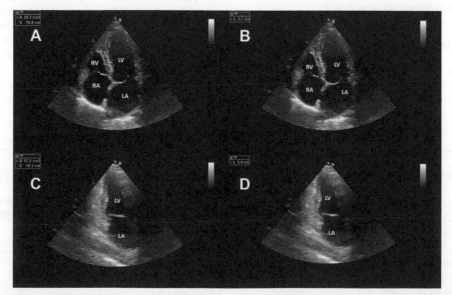

Fig. 2. LA volume, calculated by area-length method in apical 4-chamber (*A*, *B*) and 2-chamber views (*C*, *D*).

apical 4-chamber view. It can be measured (1) peak systolic (S) velocity, (2) peak anterograde diastolic (D) velocity, (3) peak retrograde diastolic (Ar) velocity, and (4) its duration during LA contraction.

Pulsed wave DMI is performed in the apical views to acquire mitral annular velocities. Measurements include the systolic (S), early diastolic (E'), and late diastolic (A') velocities. The peak velocity in late diastole secondary to atrial contraction (A') measured using pulsed wave Doppler tissue imaging is a rapid and an accurate marker of atrial function.[17]

Recently, alternative methods have been developed to measure myocardial deformation properties both by DMI-derived strain and by speckle tracking ECG strain, to detect early functional remodeling before the occurrence of anatomic alterations.

Atrial myocardial deformation properties are expressed by a dimensionless parameter, the strain that is defined as the percentage change from the original dimension, and the strain rate that is the rate of myocardial deformation and measures the velocity with which myocardial deformation occurs.[18,19] Two-dimensional strain uses grayscale imaging and is based on frame by frame tracking of small rectangular image blocks with a stable speckle pattern.[18,19] By tracing the endocardial contour on an end-systolic cavitary frame after defining the thickness of the region to be considered, the software will automatically track the atrial wall on subsequent frames.

Using this technique, analysis is performed from the 4-chamber and 2-chamber apical views regional strain of LA septum, LA lateral wall, LA inferior wall, and LA anterior wall are measured and then are averaged (see **Fig. 1**).

LEFT ATRIAL DIAMETER IN ATHLETES

Pelliccia and colleagues[4] analyzed a large population of 1777 competitive athletes, free of structural disease. The LA anteroposterior dimension was 23 to 50 mm (mean 37 ± 4 mm) in men and 20 to 46 mm (mean 32 ± 4 mm) in women. It was enlarged (ie, transverse dimension ≥40 mm) in 347 athletes (20%), including 38 (2%) with marked dilation (≥45 mm). Therefore, enlarged LA dimension greater than or equal to 40 mm was relatively common (20%), with the upper limits of 45 mm in women and 50 mm in men, distinguishing physiologic cardiac remodeling, typical of athlete's heart, from pathologic cardiac conditions. In addition, only 0.3% of those athletes with enlarged LA on initial evaluation developed a supraventricular tachycardia during the average 7-year follow-up period.

As a result, enlarged LA size (>40 mm) is relatively common in athletes and can be defined as the upper range of LA diameters (**Table 1**) to distinguish physiologic consequences of athlete's heart from primary pathologic hearth disease.[4,16]

LEFT ATRIAL VOLUME INDEX IN ATHLETES

In the athlete's heart, a mild enlargement of left atrial volume index (LAVi) is relatively common and may be considered as a physiologic adaptation to exercise conditioning.[3,5]

D'Andrea and colleagues[3] analyzed 615 consecutive elite athletes (370 endurance vs 245 strength-trained athletes, 385 men, 28.4 ± 10.2 years, range 18–40 years) who underwent a comprehensive transthoracic ECG examination. LA maximal volume was measured at the point of mitral valve opening using the biplane area-length method and corrected for body surface area. LA mild dilatation was defined as a LAVi between 29 and 33 mL/m², whereas a moderate dilatation corresponded to a LAVi greater than or equal to 34 mL/m². LAVi was mildly enlarged in 150 athletes (24.3%) and moderately enlarged only in 20, all male athletes (3.2%). Mild mitral regurgitation was observed in 64 athletes (10.3%). LAVi was significantly greater in endurance athletes (P<.01). In the overall population, the most powerful independent determinants of LAVi were type and duration of training and LV end-diastolic volume (see **Table 1**).

Table 1
Athlete's left atrial morphologic and functional parameters

Authors	Number of Athletes	Type of Sport	Parameter	Mean Value	Upper Limit
Pelliccia et al,[4] 2005	1777	Endurance or power	LA diameter (male) (mm)	37	50
			LA diameter (female) (mm)	32	45
D'Andrea et al,[3] 2010	650	Endurance or power	LA volume index (male) (mL/m²)	28	36
			LA volume index (female) (mL/m²)	26.5	33
D'Andrea et al,[5] 2008	80	Power	LA strain (%)	50	80

Nistri and colleagues[20] analyzed the relative role of multiple determinants of LAVi in athletes and nonathletes. LV end-diastolic volume index, age, and LV mass index were predictors of LAVi in both groups. Body mass index and E/A ratio were additional predictors of LAVi only in nonathletes.[16]

Recently, D'Ascenzi and colleagues[21] assessed atrial remodeling in 24 top female athletes. LAVi (24.0 ± 3.6 vs 26.7 ± 6.9 mL/m^2; P<.001) significantly increased after training in female athletes. LA global peak atrial longitudinal strain and peak atrial contraction strain significantly decreased after training in female athletes (43.9 ± 9.5% vs 39.8 ± 6.5%; P<.05 and 15.5 ± 4.0% vs 13.9 ± 4.0%; P<.05, respectively). Neither biventricular E/A ratio nor biatrial stiffness changed after training, suggesting that biatrial remodeling occurs in a model of volume rather than pressure overload.

During ventricular diastole, the LA is exposed to the LV pressure; consequently, when LV stiffness or pressure increases, LA pressure rises to maintain adequate LV filling, leading to chamber dilatation and stretch of the atrial myocardium. Therefore, LA enlargement in highly trained athletes can be considered a physiologic consequence of chronic and intensive exercise conditioning and can be included in the context of athlete's heart.

LEFT ATRIAL MYOCARDIAL FUNCTION IN ATHLETES

Atrial function is an integral part of cardiac function, important for adequate LV filling. Recognition of the upper limits of atrial function in competitive athletes may be of clinical relevance by assisting in distinguishing cardiac remodeling in athletes from structural heart disease.[3]

D'Andrea and colleagues[5] investigated, for the first time, whether mechanical dysfunction in the LA is present in patients with either physiologic or pathologic LVH, using 2-dimensional strain rate imaging. Atrial longitudinal strain was performed from the apical views for the basal segments of the LA septum, lateral wall, and roof. LA diameter and maximum volume were increased but similar between the 2 groups of subjects with LVH. LA active emptying volume and fraction were both higher in subjects with hypertension. Conversely, peak systolic myocardial atrial strain was significantly reduced in patients with pathologic LVH compared with controls and athletes for all the analyzed atrial segments (P<.0001). Using multivariate analysis, LV end-diastolic volume per body surface area (β coefficient = 0.52; P<.0001) and LV mass (β = 0.48; P = .001) in

athletes emerged as the only independent determinants of LA lateral wall peak systolic strain. In contrast, in subjects with hypertension, an independent negative association of LA lateral wall peak systolic strain with both LV mass (β = 20.42; P<.001) and circumferential end-systolic stress (β = 20.43; P<.001) was found. In addition, in the overall population of patients with LVH, LA lateral wall systolic strain (β = 0.49; P<.0001) was a powerful independent predictor of maximum workload during exercise testing.

Therefore, LA myocardial deformation assessed by strain is normal in elite athletes compared with age-matched sedentary controls and hypertensive patients, and is closely associated with functional capacity during effort.

CLINICAL IMPACT: ATRIAL FIBRILLATION IN ATHLETES

AF is the most common sustained arrhythmia in clinical practice, with a prevalence of 0.4% to 1% in the general population and increases to 8% in those older than 80 years.[22]

There is growing evidence that long-term endurance exercise may increase the risk of developing AF in the middle-aged population. Moreover, endurance training is related to the onset of lone AF, commonly defined as any AF in patients 60-years-old or younger without clinical or echocardiographic evidence of any cardiopulmonary disease, including hypertension.[23]

Numerous studies reported the correlation between long-term endurance sport practice and AF.

Karjalainen and colleagues[24] were the first in 1998 to publish a longitudinal prospective study, establishing the relationship between endurance sport practice and AF; after 10 years of follow-up, AF incidence among orienteers was 5.3%, compared with 0.9% among the control subjects.

Molina and colleagues[25] analyzed the incidence of AF in male athletes according to sport practice; the annual incidence rate of AF was 0.43 per 100 and 0.11 per 100, respectively, in a group of marathon runners and a population of sedentary men.

Finally, the Grup Integrat de Recerca en Fibrillacio Auricular (GIRAFA) studied a series of 107 consecutive subjects younger than 65 years, seen in the emergency room for an episode of LAF of less than 48 hours and a group of 107 healthy volunteers matched for age and sex were recruited as controls. Total hours and intensity of physical activity were identified with a detailed and validated questionnaire. AF was paroxysmal in 57% and persistent in the remaining 43%. Subjects with AF performed more hours of both moderate and heavy intensity physical activity.[26]

In contrast to these previous studies, Pelliccia and colleagues[4] studied the long-term arrhythmic consequences of LA enlargement in 1777 competitive athletes (71% of whom were male), free of structural cardiovascular disease that were participating in 38 different sports. They reported a low incidence of AF and other supraventricular tachyarrhythmias (prevalence <1%) and similar to that in the general population of comparable age and sex, despite the frequency of LA enlargement. However, in contrast to previous studies showing an association between AF and long-term endurance sport practice, the population analyzed by Pelliccia and colleagues[4] were young athletes (mean age 24 ± 6 years) involved in vigorous training programs for a mean time of only 6 years, studied at the moment of their highest activity.

On the other hand, Mozaffarian and colleagues,[27] in the Cardiovascular Health Study, showed that light to moderate physical activities, such as leisure-time activity and walking, were associated with significantly lower AF incidence in older adults (>65 years old), but this was not true with high-intensity exercise. Thus, a U-shaped dose-response curve can be inferred, suggesting that regular mild to moderate exercise may provide a degree of protection from AF, whereas more sustained vigorous exertion represents a risk factor.[27]

Finally, the clinical profile of sport-related AF is a middle-aged male athlete with a history of long-term regular endurance sport practice, currently involved in high endurance training. The AF is usually paroxysmal, initially self-limited, and progressively increasing in duration. Typically, AF episodes occur at night or after meals, revealing that AF may be related to increased vagal tone[28–30] (Fig. 3).

Various pathophysiological mechanisms are responsible for the increased risk of AF in athletes. Winhelm and colleagues[31] analyzed 492 marathoners and found an enlarged LA in 24% of runners in the low training group (<1500 h of lifetime training), 40% of runners in the medium training group (1500–4500 h), and 83% of runners in the high training group (>4500 h), demonstrating a relationship between dimension of LA and hours of lifetime training.

Other mechanisms responsible of development of AF in athletes are atrial ectopic beats, influence of the autonomic nervous system with increased vagal tone, fibrosis with collagen deposition, inflammation with activation of circulating monocytes, and production of proinflammatory cytokines.[32–34]

LA diameter and long-standing AF are the principal independent predictors of clinical recurrence. After a successful ablation procedure

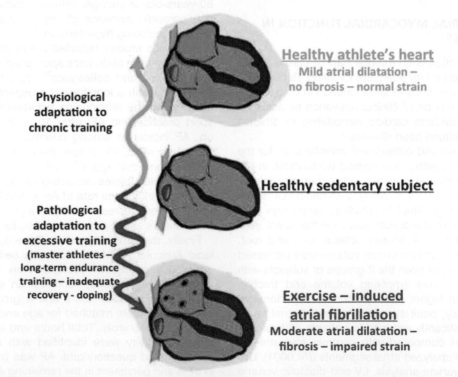

Physiological adaptation to chronic training

Healthy athlete's heart
Mild atrial dilatation –
no fibrosis – normal strain

Healthy sedentary subject

Pathological adaptation to excessive training (master athletes – long-term endurance training – inadequate recovery - doping)

Exercise – induced atrial fibrillation
Moderate atrial dilatation –
fibrosis – impaired strain

Fig. 3. Different models of LA remodeling to exercise: physiologic (*green arrow*) and pathologic adaptation (*red arrow*). (Illustration by Germano Massenzio, Naples, Italy.)

without symptomatic recurrence for 3 months, return to sport activity is warranted, with a close follow-up of athletes every 6 months.[30–35]

CARDIAC MAGNETIC RESONANCE AND LEFT ATRIAL MORPHOLOGY IN ATHLETES

Cardiac magnetic resonance (CMR) has the capability of acquiring tomographic images of the hypertrophied LV chamber, with tissue contrast and border definition that are often superior to that achievable with ECG. In addition, the LA and pulmonary veins can be readily imaged using standard techniques, and contrast-enhanced magnetic resonance angiography, as well as high-resolution late gadolinium enhancement, provides greater anatomic detail and information about the presence of scar in LA walls, even after radiofrequency ablation.

Little data exist by CMR on atrial adaptation to training. As expected, atrial volumes were significantly larger in athletes.[36] However, atrial volumes normalized for total heart volume did not differ between athletes and controls, indicating a balanced enlargement. There was only a small difference between female controls and female athletes, suggesting that atrial adjustment to training is more modest in women.

SUMMARY

In large populations of highly trained athletes, mild LA enlargement is relatively common and may be identified as a physiologic adaptation to exercise conditioning. LA remodeling is associated with a higher risk of AF, especially in middle-aged men athletes, with a history of intensive long-term endurance training. However, the absolute risk of this arrhythmia among sport practitioners remains low and mild physical activities, such as leisure-time activity and walking, are associated with significantly lower AF incidence in older adults. Finally, AF in athletes is not associated with an increased risk of death because sport activity has important cardiovascular benefits and reduces other risk factors, with a lower prevalence of hypertension, diabetes mellitus, and coronary artery disease in athlete's population.

Taken together, these findings point out the need for including LA measurement in the echocardiographic assessment of athletes, referring to normal reference values. Whereas mild to moderate LA enlargement can be considered a physiologic adaptation of training, severe LA dilation should raise suspicion on the coexistence of cardiac disease and lead to further diagnostic investigation (**Fig. 4**).

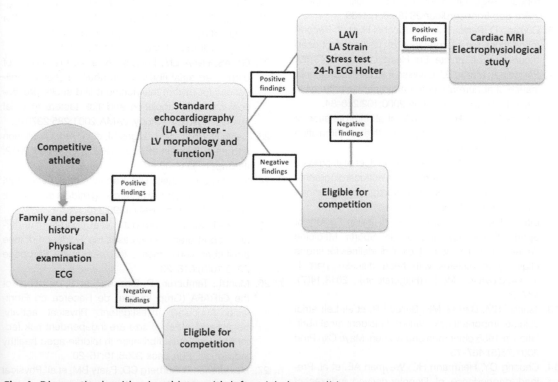

Fig. 4. Diagnostic algorithm in athletes with left atrial abnormalities.

REFERENCES

1. Ancona R, Comenale Pinto S, Caso P, et al. Left atrium by echocardiography in clinical practice: from conventional methods to new echocardiographic techniques. ScientificWorldJournal 2014; 2014:451042.
2. D'Andrea A, Riegler L, Rucco MA, et al. Left atrial volume index in healthy subjects: clinical and echocardiographic correlates. Echocardiography 2013; 30:1001–7.
3. D'Andrea A, Riegler L, Cocchia R, et al. Left atrial volume index in highly trained athletes. Am Heart J 2010;159(6):1155–61.
4. Pelliccia A, Maron BJ, Di Paolo FM, et al. Prevalence and clinical significance of left atrial remodeling in competitive athletes. J Am Coll Cardiol 2005;46(4): 690–6.
5. D'Andrea A, De Corato G, Scarafile R, et al. Left atrial myocardial function in either physiological or pathological left ventricular hypertrophy: a two-dimensional speckle strain study. Br J Sports Med 2008;42(8):696–702.
6. Mont L, Sambola A, Brugada J, et al. Long-lasting sport practice and lone atrial fibrillation. Eur Heart J 2002;23(6):477–82.
7. Lang RM, Badano LP, Mor-Avi V, et al. Recommendations for cardiac chamber quantification by echocardiography in adults: an update from the American Society of Echocardiography and the European Association of Cardiovascular Imaging. J Am Soc Echocardiogr 2015;28(1):1–39.
8. Corrado D, Pelliccia A, Heidbuchel H, et al. Recommendations for interpretation of 12-lead electrocardiogram in the athlete. Eur Heart J 2010;31:243–59.
9. Pelliccia A, Maron BJ, Culasso F, et al. Clinical significance of abnormal electrocardiographic patterns in trained athletes. Circulation 2000;102:278–84.
10. Uberoi A, Stein R, Perez MV, et al. Interpretation of the electrocardiogram of young athletes. Circulation 2011;124(6):746–57.
11. Brosnan M, La Gerche A, Kalman J, et al. Comparison of frequency of significant electrocardiographic abnormalities in endurance versus nonendurance athletes. Am J Cardiol 2014;113(9):1567–73.
12. Biffi A, Delise P, Zeppilli P, et al, Italian Society of Sports Cardiology and Italian Sports Medicine Federation. Italian cardiological guidelines for sports eligibility in athletes with heart disease: part 1. J Cardiovasc Med (Hagerstown) 2013;14(7): 477–99.
13. Tsang TSM, Barnes ME, Bailey KR, et al. Left atrial volume: important risk marker of incident atrial fibrillation in 1655 older men and women. Mayo Clin Proc 2001;76(5):467–75.
14. Choong CY, Herrmann HC, Weyman AE, et al. Pre-load dependence of Doppler-derived indexes of left ventricular diastolic function in humans. J Am Coll Cardiol 1987;10(4):800–8.
15. Prioli A, Marino P, Lanzoni L, et al. Increasing degrees of left ventricular filling impairment modulate left atrial function in humans. Am J Cardiol 1998; 82(6):756–61.
16. Galderisi M, Cardim N, D'Andrea A, et al. The multi-modality cardiac imaging approach to the Athlete's heart: an expert consensus of the European Association of Cardiovascular Imaging. Eur Heart J Cardiovasc Imaging 2015;16:353.
17. Hesse B, Schuele SU, Thamilasaran M, et al. A rapid method to quantify left atrial contractile function: Doppler tissue imaging of the mitral annulus during atrial systole. Eur J Echocardiogr 2004;5(1):86–92.
18. Inaba Y, Yuda S, Kobayashi N, et al. Strain rate imaging for noninvasive functional quantification of the left atrium: comparative studies in controls and patients with atrial fibrillation. J Am Soc Echocardiogr 2005;18(7):729–36.
19. D'Andrea A, Caso P, Romano S, et al. Different effects of cardiac resynchronization therapy on left atrial function in patients with either idiopathic or ischaemic dilated cardiomyopathy: a two-dimensional speckle strain study. Eur Heart J 2007;28(22):2738–48.
20. Nistri S, Galderisi M, Ballo P, et al, Working Group on Echocardiography of the Italian Society of Cardiology. Determinants of echocardiographic left atrial volume: implications for normalcy. Eur J Echocardiogr 2011;12(11):826–33.
21. D'Ascenzi F, Pelliccia A, Natali BM, et al. Morphological and functional adaptation of left and right atria induced by training in highly trained female athletes. Circ Cardiovasc Imaging 2014;7(2):222–9.
22. Go AS, Hylek EM, Phillips KA, et al. Prevalence of diagnosed atrial fibrillation in adults: national implications for rhythm management and stroke prevention: the anticoagulation and risk factors in atrial fibrillation (ATRIA) Study. JAMA 2001;285:2370–5.
23. Calvo N, Brugada J, Sitges M, et al. Atrial fibrillation and atrial flutter in athletes. Br J Sports Med 2012; 46(Suppl 1):i37–43.
24. Karjalainen J, Kujala UM, Kaprio J, et al. Lone atrial fibrillation in vigorously exercising middle aged men: case-control study. BMJ 1998;316:1784–5.
25. Molina L, Mont L, Marrugat J, et al. Long-term endurance sport practice increases the incidence of lone atrial fibrillation in men: a follow-up study. Europace 2008;10(5):618–23.
26. Mont L, Tamborero D, Elosua R, et al, on behalf of the GIRAFA (Grup Integrat de Recerca en Fibrillacio Auricular) Investigators. Physical activity, height and left atrial size are independent risk factors for lone atrial fibrillation in middle-aged healthy individuals. Europace 2008;10:15–20.
27. Mozaffarian D, Furberg CD, Psaty BM, et al. Physical activity and incidence of atrial fibrillation in older

adults. The cardiovascular health study. Circulation 2008;118:800–7.

28. La Gerche A, Schmied CM. Atrial fibrillation in athletes and the interplay between exercise and health. Eur Heart J 2013;34(47):3599–602.

29. Mont L, Elosua R, Brugada J. Endurance sport practice as a risk factor for atrial fibrillation and atrial flutter. Europace 2009;11(1):11–7.

30. Hoogsteen J, Schep G, van Hemel NM, et al. Paroxysmal atrial fibrillation in male endurance athletes. A 9-year follow up. Europace 2004;6:222–8.

31. Winhelm M, Roten L, Tanner H, et al. Atrial remodeling, autonomic tone, and lifetime training hours in nonelite athletes. Am J Cardiol 2011;108:580–5.

32. Furlanello F, Bertoldi A, Dallago M, et al. Atrial fibrillation in elite athletes. J Cardiovasc Electrophysiol 1998;9:S63–8.

33. Lindsay MM, Dunn FG. Biochemical evidence of myocardial fibrosis in veteran endurance athletes. Br J Sports Med 2007;41:447–52.

34. Aviles R, Martin D, Apperson-Hansen C, et al. Inflammation as a risk factor for atrial fibrillation. Circulation 2003;108:3006–10.

35. Heidbuchel H, Panhuyzen-Goedkoop N, Corrado D, et al. Recommendations for participation in leisure-time physical activity and competitive sports in patients with arrhythmias and potentially arrhythmogenic conditions Part I: supraventricular arrhythmias and pacemakers. Eur J Cardiovasc Prev Rehabil 2006;13:475–84.

36. Mosén H, Steding-Ehrenborg K. Atrial remodelling is less pronounced in female endurance-trained athletes compared with that in male athletes. Scand Cardiovasc J 2014;48(1):20–6.

Atrial Fibrillation in Endurance Athletes
From Mechanism to Management

Adrian D. Elliott, PhD*, Rajiv Mahajan, MD, PhD,
Dennis H. Lau, MBBS, PhD, Prashanthan Sanders, MBBS, PhD

KEYWORDS

• Atrial fibrillation • Athlete • Arrhythmia • Exercise • Cardiac

KEY POINTS

• Atrial fibrillation (AF) risk is elevated by endurance sports participation. Risk estimates range from a 3-fold to 9-fold increase, based on smaller case-control studies, to a 30% increase, based on larger cohort studies.
• Atrial remodeling seems to be a primary mechanistic promoter of AF in athletes, likely accompanied by autonomic alterations favoring re-entry.
• Despite limited data in athletes, treatment options include radiofrequency catheter ablation, which has been shown to have similar efficacy to that in nonathletic control patients. Rate control may be poorly tolerated, whereas anticoagulation should be guided by recommended guidelines using the CHA_2DS_2-VASc score.

INTRODUCTION

Exercise training exerts considerable health benefits, contributing to a substantial decline in cardiac and all-cause mortality in those who engage in regular physical activity.[1] Both measured physical activity[2] and cardiorespiratory fitness[3] strongly predict long-term health outcomes. In those who engage in more extensive endurance training, the benefits on mortality are profound,[4] although not necessarily over and above those observed with more modest exercise habits.

Despite the stream of empirical evidence supporting the benefits of exercise, the concept of exercise producing adverse effects on the heart draws considerable interest from both the medical research environment and the wider population. Traditional and social media are drawn to the stories in which an athlete experiences a cardiac disorder or worse, sudden cardiac death.

Although these events are infrequent and isolated,[5,6] there is mounting evidence to suggest that prolonged exercise training over many years

Disclosures: Dr P. Sanders reports having served on the advisory board of Biosense-Webster, Medtronic, CathRx, and St Jude Medical. Dr P. Sanders reports having received lecture and consulting fees from Biosense Webster, Medtronic, St. Jude Medical, and Boston Scientific. Dr P. Sanders reports having received research funding from Medtronic, St Jude Medical, Boston Scientific, Biotronik, and Sorin. The other authors report no conflicts.
Sources of Funding: Dr R. Mahajan is supported by the Leo J. Mahar Lectureship from the University of Adelaide and by an Early Career Fellowship jointly funded by the National Health and Medical Research Council of Australia and the National Heart Foundation of Australia. Dr D.H. Lau is supported by a Robert J. Craig Lectureship from the University of Adelaide. Dr P. Sanders is supported by a Practitioner Fellowship from the National Health and Medical Research Council of Australia and by the National Heart Foundation of Australia.
Centre for Heart Rhythm Disorders, South Australian Health and Medical Research Institute, Royal Adelaide Hospital, University of Adelaide, Adelaide, South Australia, Australia
* Corresponding author. Centre for Heart Rhythm Disorders, Level 8, South Australian Health and Medical Research Institute, Royal Adelaide Hospital, University of Adelaide, Adelaide, South Australia 5000, Australia.
E-mail address: adrian.elliott@adelaide.edu.au

0733-8651/16/© 2016 Elsevier Inc. All rights reserved.

may result in ventricular arrhythmias for a small minority of athletes.[7] Yet, more common within the endurance athlete population, with consistent data from both Europe and the United States, is the relative increase in atrial arrhythmia risk in endurance athletes compared with nonathletes.

PREVALENCE OF ATRIAL ARRHYTHMIAS IN ENDURANCE ATHLETES

Atrial fibrillation (AF) is the most common clinical arrhythmia with a growing global burden[8] leading to rising hospitalizations and health care demands.[9–11] Risk factors for AF include hypertension, obesity, and diabetes mellitus, as well as obstructive sleep apnea and alcohol intake. Recent evidence strongly supports risk factor modification, including increasing cardiorespiratory fitness, for the management of AF.[12–14] However, in the past 20 years, there has been a swell of evidence confirming that endurance sports practice also presents an independent risk factor for AF.

Based on the clinical observation that AF appeared more frequently in endurance athletes, Karjalainen and colleagues[15] compared AF prevalence in highly ranked orienteers versus age-matched healthy control participants from an earlier study. Using self-report to identify participants with AF before confirmation by medical records, AF was found to be more prevalent in athletes versus nonathletes (5.3% vs 0.9%, relative risk 5.5, 95% CI 1.3–24.4), despite lower mortality and vascular events in the athletes. In a case analysis, Mont and colleagues[16] later revealed that among lone AF patients seen in an outpatient arrhythmia clinic, the proportion of athletes among the AF group was substantially greater than that in the general population (63% v 15%, respectively). The same center subsequently published the findings of an age-matched case-control study,[17] in which 51 men with lone AF were compared against controls selected from the general population. The proportion of lone AF subjects reporting current sports practice was higher than in controls (31% v 14%; odds ratio [OR] 3.1, 95% CI 1.4–7.1). Interestingly, this study also attempted to determine a dose-risk assessment using sporting history questionnaires. Current sporting practice with greater than 1500 lifetime exercise hours increased AF risk (OR 2.9, 95% CI 1.2–6.9) compared with those who did not engage in sports. More recently, a similar case control study of subjects with lone AF has revealed a threshold of 2000 lifetime training hours, above which AF risk increases (OR 3.88, 95% CI: 1.55–9.73).[18]

Similar conclusions have been drawn from studies comparing AF prevalence within an athletic population compared with sedentary controls. Molina and colleagues[19] compared 183 amateur marathon runners with a population-based sample of 290 sedentary controls. The annual incidence rate of AF was significantly higher in athletes versus sedentary controls (0.43/100 persons vs 0.11/100 persons, adjusted hazard ratio 8.8, 95% CI: 1.3–61.3). Also in runners, Wilhelm and colleagues[20] noted an AF prevalence of 6.7% for athletes with a mean age of 42 years, considerably higher than recent estimates that suggest the prevalence for 40 to 44 year old men in Western Europe is approximately 0.2%.[8] In a comparison of former professional cyclists versus age and gender-matched golfers, Baldesberger and colleagues[21] identified 6 cases (10%) of AF or atrial flutter in the 62 cyclists, compared with 0 cases from the 62 participant control group.

One of the primary limitations with these studies is the relatively small sample size. This has been addressed recently by a series of studies from Scandinavia in which larger cohorts have been assessed to address the AF risk associated with endurance exercise. In more than 52,000 participants of the Vasaloppet 90 km cross-country ski race between 1989 and 1998, AF occurred more frequently in those who had completed greater than 5 races compared with those who had completed only 1 race, albeit with a lower risk estimate than shown previously (hazard ratio 1.29).[22] In this population, the number of completed races was taken as a surrogate measure of total training dose, although the reference group included participants who had completed 1 race, rather than a true sedentary group. This subtlety likely dampens the true risk estimate drawn from this study, although it does confirm the increased frequency of arrhythmias in athletes. Additionally, Myrstad and colleagues[23] compared a sample of cross-country skiers to a group recruited from a large population survey study. This study of more than 3500 participants (mean age ~65 y) found that participants with greater than 30 years of endurance training practice were at a greater risk of both atrial flutter and AF. The prevalence of self-report AF was 12.5% in athletes, with an adjusted risk increase of 26% (OR 1.26) for lone AF per each 10-year increase in training history.

Taken together, these studies provide convincing evidence that endurance exercise training leads to an elevated risk of AF that may be more pronounced in those athletes with more extensive exercise training history.

Searching for a Common Definition

Establishing a link between exercise training and AF depends strongly on the definition of what is considered as training rather than general physical activity. Similarly, classifying an individual as an athlete may be subjective. Studies have addressed the relationship by classifying athletes using methods such as those who participate in endurance competition,[19,22] former professional athletes,[21] current sports ranking,[15] and self-reported lifetime training hours assessed by questionnaire.[18,24] Between-study methodological differences present an important confounder, particularly when trying to elucidate a threshold above which AF risk is exaggerated. Recent trends in exercise monitoring using mobile devices and wearable technologies will enable prospective studies to provide more objective measures of training status and a more precise description of the association between exercise and AF.

MECHANISMS IN THE PATHOGENESIS OF ATRIAL FIBRILLATION IN ATHLETES

The pathophysiological mechanisms leading to the development of AF are complex and vary between individuals but commonly involve structural, electrical, and autonomic remodeling of the atria, predisposing to re-entry or triggered activity (**Fig. 1**).[25]

In animal models of hypertension,[26] obstructive sleep apnea,[27] and obesity,[28] extensive electrophysiological and structural remodeling, including decreased conduction velocity and atrial voltages, increased conduction heterogeneity, fractionated electrograms, and fibrosis, leads to heightened AF susceptibility. Although traditional risk factors such as obesity and hypertension are strong predictors of AF within the general population, the burden of these risk factors in an athlete population is low. The mechanisms of AF promotion in endurance athletes is not well understood but potentially includes atrial enlargement, vagal enhancement, and increased inflammation as primary mediators.

Atrial Structural Remodeling

Biatrial dilation is a common, well-described adaptation within the athlete's heart.[20,29] Left and right atria undergo enlargement as a result of exercise training, although the clinical significance of such changes is to be determined. In 1777 competitive athletes, left atrial dilation occurred in 20% of athletes but was not associated with increased arrhythmia prevalence.[30] This was a cross-sectional analysis of a young athletic cohort (mean age 24 ± 6 y) that identified arrhythmia by symptoms and routine electrocardiogram, thus raising the possibility that asymptomatic episodes

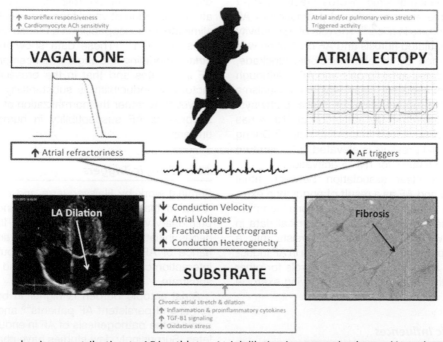

Fig. 1. The mechanisms contributing to AF in athletes. Atrial dilation is commonly observed in endurance athletes and may accompany atrial fibrosis, contributing to a vulnerable substrate. Vagal tone is elevated following the onset of exercise training and may promote re-entry by shortening of the effective refractory period. Increased atrial ectopy has been reported in some studies and may precede the onset of AF in some athletes. ACh, acetylcholine; LA, left atrium; TGF, transforming growth factor.

may have been overlooked. Case-control and cohort studies with an older population support left atrial size as an independent predictor of AF.[19,31]

Fibrosis is a common feature of atrial remodeling observed with other risk factors, such as hypertension[26] and obesity,[28] and may feature within the atria of well-trained endurance athletes. Fibrosis within the ventricles of endurance athletes has been demonstrated previously,[32,33] although, to the authors' knowledge, there are little data on fibrosis within the atrial walls.

In rat models of marathon running, exercise-induced remodeling, including both atrial and ventricular fibrosis, has been demonstrated, consequently contributing to an increased susceptibility for AF[34] and ventricular tachycardia.[35] The profibrotic process is enhanced by several signaling pathways, including the renin-angiotensin-aldosterone system, transforming growth factor-β_1, connective tissue growth factor, proinflammatory cytokines, and oxidative stress.[36] Endurance exercise is associated with acute postexercise elevations in both inflammation and oxidative stress,[37,38] repeated bouts of which may contribute to collagen deposition within the atrial walls.

Animal studies have confirmed the role of inflammation for exercise-induced atrial fibrosis; pharmacologic inhibition of tumor necrosis factor (TNF)-α abolished the exercise-induced promotion of AF and atrial fibrosis in mice.[39] The role of p38 activity in TNF-α regulated fibrosis and AF promotion was also confirmed by its pharmacologic blockade, which prevented atrial fibrosis and AF.[39] Although it is not immediately clear which mechanisms contribute to upregulation of these pathways, the role of stretch in the activation of TNF-α has been shown previously in cardiac cells.[40] During exercise, atrial pressure is elevated,[41,42] therefore providing a stimulus for TNF-α activation.

Despite a clear association between atrial remodeling and AF as a result of endurance exercise, atrial dilation and fibrosis alone seem to be insufficient to promote AF. Preclinical data in rats[34] show that atrial fibrosis persists into a detraining period despite a regression in AF inducibility. This key finding supports the role for other factors in the promotion of AF following exercise training.

Autonomic Influences

Well-trained athletes exhibit enhanced measures of vagal tone, such as heart rate variability,[43] relative to nonathletes. Vagal tone favors a reduced refractoriness and enhanced excitability of the myocardium.[44] In addition, it potentially creates the milieu for re-entry within the atria, leading to AF.[45] Indeed, Bettoni and Zimmermann[46] reported on autonomic variations, from adrenergic drive through an abrupt shift toward vagal dominance, immediately preceding AF initiation. Enhanced vagal tone reduces effective refractory periods within the atria via acetylcholine-mediated K^+ currents, thus potentially contributing to the increased observation of vagally mediated lone AF in endurance athletes.[17] Furthermore, vagally mediated bradycardia would be expected to aggravate the impact of atrial stretch, structural remodeling, and potentially provides a more vulnerable period during which triggers can capture the atrial myocardium.

Preclinical data support a vagal mechanistic involvement in the AF observed in athletes. Guasch and colleagues[34] demonstrated enhanced vagal tone following 16 weeks of training in rats, despite no alterations in sympathetic drive. Moreover, vagal tone was reversible and was indistinguishable between trained and sedentary rats following detraining. Most notably, vagal enhancement was temporally associated with AF inducibility in the trained group, therefore portraying a central role for autonomic alterations as a mechanistic contributor to the AF promotion by exercise. More recently, conflicting data from further preclinical data suggest a lesser role for autonomic alterations; inhibition of vagal tone reduced but did not eliminate AF susceptibility in a mouse model of exercise training.[39] These data show that parallel atrial remodeling and vagal enhancement promote AF in athletes and that in the presence of both factors AF inducibility is substantially increased. However, whether the normalization of vagal tone suppresses AF susceptibility in humans is still unclear.

Atrial Ectopic Triggers

Seminal work by Haïssaguerre and colleagues[47] revealed that ectopic beats originating from the pulmonary veins commonly leads to the spontaneous initiation of AF. The initiation and maintenance of AF can therefore be attributed to the interaction of a trigger, modulator, and vulnerable substrate.

Atrial ectopic burden is higher in both paroxysmal and persistent AF patients[48] and may play a role in the pathogenesis of AF in endurance athletes. Surprisingly, few studies have characterized atrial ectopic burden in endurance athletes. In former professional cyclists, atrial ectopic burden was not significantly higher than a control group matched by age and gender, despite higher prevalence of AF.[21] In contrast, male runners with a training history greater than 4500 lifetime hours had significantly higher atrial ectopic burden compared with those with less than 1500 training hours.[20] However, the mean burden of ectopic beats was lower than that reported in subjects with AF.[48] It remains unclear whether exercise training per se results in a clinically significant increase in atrial ectopy that contributes to the development of AF in endurance athletes.

MANAGEMENT OF ATRIAL FIBRILLATION IN ATHLETES
Evaluation of an Athlete with Atrial Fibrillation

The initial evaluation of an athlete with confirmed or suspected AF should seek to exclude structural or electrical abnormalities. Evaluation for coronary artery disease should be considered in the older athlete. In addition, the clinician needs to consider the possibility of inherited channelopathies and the potential existence of conventional cardiovascular risk factors. Dilated cardiomyopathies, hypertrophic cardiomyopathy, and valvular abnormalities should be excluded by echocardiography. An electrocardiogram will permit the assessment of accessory pathways, conduction abnormalities, and channelopathies that may contribute to the onset of AF. The risk of AF is increased in those with channelopathies such as Brugada, short QT, and long QT syndromes; with these conditions conferring additional risks in athletes. In particular, AF may be the first arrhythmogenic presentation of these conditions and therefore requires consideration. Similarly, evaluation for conventional cardiovascular risk factors, such as obstructive sleep apnea, hypertension, type II diabetes mellitus, hyperlipidemia, alcohol intake, and hyperthyroidism, should be undertaken. Many of these risk factors have a low prevalence in an athletic population; however, may be present in some and should be considered in the older athlete. Prolonged or frequent rhythm monitoring may be necessary to evaluate the frequency and burden of AF, as well as characterize any asymptomatic episodes.

Despite an absence of detailed decision-making guidelines for the management of AF in athletes, current American Heart Association and American College of Cardiology (AHA/ACC) guidelines regarding eligibility and disqualification recommendations for competitive athletes with cardiovascular abnormalities[49] supports continued sports participation in athletes with well-tolerated, self-terminating AF or AF that is appropriately managed (**Table 1**).

Detraining

In animal studies, detraining reverses the AF susceptibility brought about by long-term, intensive exercise training,[34] although fibrosis remains elevated within the atria. There are few data on the role of detraining in human athletes with AF, although there are isolated reports of its efficacy for the management of AF before the return to sports participation.[50] In athletes with confirmed or borderline left ventricular hypertrophy, detraining has been shown to reduce atrial dimensions in some studies[51] but not others,[52] although between-studies differences may be due to different baseline left atrial dimension.[51] How this translates for the athlete with AF is not immediately clear but the rationale for detraining presumably centers on a regression in the underlying proarrhythmogenic substrate or a normalization of autonomic influences. In the presence of marked bradycardia, which in this population most often is related to vagal nerve remodeling and altered sinus node function,[53,54] detraining can be associated with an improvement in heart rates,[52] potentially reducing the period during which the atrial myocardium is vulnerable to triggered activity.

Importantly, the feasibility of detraining depends on the athlete's competitive situation in which a professional athlete is unlikely to favor such an approach in the long-term. Full physical deconditioning should also be considered in the context of potential adverse effects encountered by a long-term decline in physical activity levels. In cases in which a detraining strategy is agreed on following consultation with the athlete, the reduction in training load should be considered relative to the athlete's regular program. For example, in an elite endurance athlete with a training volume of greater than 25 hours per week, as shown previously,[55] a prescribed detraining strategy may target less than 5 hours per week, thus representing an 80% reduction in training load. For an athlete engaging in 5 hours per week of training, less than 2 hours per week may be more appropriate. Despite its logical rationale, there is currently no available evidence regarding the efficacy of detraining for the reduction of AF burden. Further studies are required to characterize the outcomes of detraining in athletes with AF and to define the optimal detraining strategy in which this is considered appropriate for AF management.

Rate Control

Current AHA/ACC and Heart Rhythm Society (HRS) guidelines[56] for the management of patients

Table 1
Studies reporting the outcome of catheter ablation in athletes

Study	Sample (n)	Age (y)	AF Type (% Persistent)	Athletes	Procedure	Follow-Up	Outcome (% AF-Freedom)
Furlanello et al,[63] 2008	20 A (no C)	44 ± 13	NR	Regular training + competition; >20 h per wk, mean duration 25.2 y	PVI	36 ± 13 mo	OFF AADs Single procedure: NR multiple procedures: 90% (A)
Calvo et al,[64] 2010	42 Lone AF A; 140 AF C	52 ± 10 (A); 49 ± 11 (C)	26% (A); 36% C	Regular endurance training >3 h per wk, >10 y	PVI + linear lines	19 ± 12 mo	OFF AADs Single procedure: 59% (A), 48% (C) Multiple procedures: 81% (A), 63% (C)
Koopman et al,[65] 2011	94 A; 41 C	51 ± 8 (A); 52 ± 8 (C)	13% (A); 5% (C)	Regular sports training >3 h per wk, >10 y	PVI + linear lines if required	46 ± 28 mo	With AADs Single procedure: 42% (A), 48% (C) Multiple procedures: 85% (A), 87% (C)

Abbreviations: A, athlete; AADs, antiarrhythmic drugs; C, control; NR, not reported; PVI, pulmonary vein isolation.

with AF recommend ventricular rate control for patients with paroxysmal and persistent AF. For symptomatic patients, stricter rate control (resting heart rate<80 beats per minute [bpm]) is suggested as a reasonable target, although for asymptomatic patients, a more lenient target of less than 110 bpm may be appropriate. There are no studies evaluating the efficacy and performance impact of rate control medication in athletes with atrial arrhythmias. For the athlete, beta-blockade may not be well tolerated and is likely to result in a decline in cardiovascular performance during submaximal and maximal exercise.[57,58] Furthermore, bradycardia with nocturnal pauses is also common in this cohort, which may contraindicate beta-blockade. Additional issues arise for some competitive athletes in whom beta-blockers are banned in competition. Although data are lacking, the exercise performance of athletes may be comparatively less impaired by calcium antagonists,[59] which may be a preferred option in this context.

Rate control in the athlete is notoriously vexed and poorly tolerated, predominantly due to the frequent occurrence of resting bradycardia and the impact of such rate-limiting drugs on exercise performance. Therefore, in the authors' experiences, these factors are common reasons for the early use of rhythm control strategies.

Rhythm Control

Ongoing symptoms and poor tolerability of rate control strategies provide the primary rationale for pursuing a rhythm control strategy. The effect of AF on exercise performance, particularly in young, competitive athletes, provides additional justification for prompt rhythm control, obviating rate control.

To date, there is little available evidence regarding the efficacy of antiarrhythmic drugs (AADs) for athletes with AF. Indeed, these have resulted in a similar experience to what has been observed with rate control medications; that is, they are often poorly tolerated. The most often used strategy has been the use of the class IC agents flecainide or propafenone as a pill in the pocket approach for the management of out-of-hospital, symptomatic episodes,[56,60] although this has not been specifically evaluated in athletes with AF. Caution should be noted regarding the management of AF by class IC agents given that they lower atrial rate activity, potentially organizing AF into atrial tachycardia with 1 to 1 conduction.[61] This may have specific consequences in the athlete whereby the low resting heart rate prohibits the addition of concurrent atrioventricular (AV)

nodal blocking agents during exercise, with an increase in circulating catecholamines. There may be further acceleration of AV conduction, which can more frequently result in 1 to 1 conduction of organized rhythms to the ventricle. In our patients using pill in the pocket strategy early on, we specifically instruct cessation of exercise during the period of arrhythmia and use of both an AV nodal blocking agent with a class IC agent. In an interesting subset of patients in whom arrhythmia is triggered only during exercise, we have used premedication 30 to 60 minutes before activity, with some success. In our experience, the chronic use of AADs is poorly tolerated in athletes.

The poor tolerability of pharmaceutical therapies has led to the increasing use of catheter ablation. In recent years, catheter ablation has evolved considerably with subsequent improvements in both safety and efficacy,[56,62] thus potentially reducing the dependence on rate control and anti-arrhythmic medication for the management of AF.

In the first of recent studies on the use of catheter ablation in an athletic population (**Table 2**), Furlanello and colleagues[63] reported on a cohort of 20 athletes, predominantly competing in endurance sports (>20 h/wk, mean duration of 25.2 y). Participants in this series were men with a mean age of 44 years (range 22–62 y). The ablation strategy sought pulmonary vein isolation in a first procedure, with conduction recurrence assessed in a prescheduled second procedure 3 months later. Over a 36-month follow-up without AADs, 18 (90%) of athletes remained AF-free. Importantly, both exercise tolerance and quality of life were significantly approved after catheter ablation. In the 2 athletes experiencing recurrent AF, these were short-lasting occasional episodes that were self-terminating and did not limit exercise participation or performance.

In a later series, Calvo and colleagues[64] reported on the outcomes of catheter ablation between lone AF subjects with and without a history of regular endurance sports participation (3 h/wk for at least 10 y before diagnosis). Following a 19-month follow-up, there was no significant difference between athletes and non-athletes for single-procedure arrhythmia recurrence (59% v 48%, respectively). Following multiple procedures, athletes were more likely to maintain arrhythmia-free survival than nonathletes (81 v 63%, respectively).

Similarly, the success rates of single and multiple procedure ablation was similar between athletes and nonathletes in a study by Koopman and colleagues.[65] Following a 3-year follow-up, 85% of athletes remained arrhythmia free after multiple procedures, compared with 87% in the

Table 2
Summary of available guidelines regarding atrial fibrillation in athletes

Guideline Statement	Recommendations
AHA/ACC Eligibility and Disqualification Recommendations for Competitive Athletes With Cardiovascular Abnormalities: Task Force 9: Arrhythmias and Conduction Defects[49]	1. Athletes with AF should undergo a workup that includes thyroid function tests, queries for drug use, electrocardiogram, and echocardiogram (class I; level of evidence B). 2. Athletes with low-risk AF that is well tolerated and self-terminating may participate in all competitive sports without therapy (class I; level of evidence C). 3. In athletes with AF, when antithrombotic therapy, other than aspirin, is indicated, it is reasonable to consider the bleeding risk in the context of the specific sport before clearance (class IIa; level of evidence C). 4. Catheter ablation for AF could obviate rate control or AADs and should be considered (class IIA, level of evidence B)
2014 AHA/ACC/HRS Guideline for the Management of Patients With Atrial Fibrillation[56]	No specific recommendations. However, text raises following suggestions: • Rule out hypertension and coronary artery disease in the older athlete • Consider ventricular rate response during AF episode, which may require maximal exercise testing. • Consider pill in the pocket approach or catheter ablation.

control group. Rates of arrhythmia recurrence were also similar between endurance athletes and athletes from nonendurance sports.

Several complications have been recognized with the use of catheter ablation for AF.[62] Some of these may have an impact on the performance of the athlete and may warrant specific discussion. Vascular complications at the site of venous access can limit mobility and, in the rare patient, result in pain at the site for a more prolonged period, which may limit the types of exercise that can be performed, usually limited to the first few weeks or months after ablation. Dyspnea is often observed early after the procedure and in the athlete can be noticeably more profound given the baseline level of functioning. Most often this is due to transient factors related to a fluid overload, atrial mechanical dysfunction, or local trauma to the lung. Persistent dyspnea longer than the first 3 months requires evaluation and may have longer term consequences to the level of performance. Phrenic nerve injury is a recognized complication, occurring more frequently with the use of cryoballoon ablation.[66] Although mostly these recover, the course of recovery can be quite prolonged, in rare cases persisting more than 12 months. Fixed obstructive lesions can result in a more lasting impact on exercise performance. These include pulmonary venous stenosis or rarely the stiff left atrial syndrome.[67]

Although evidence for this is sparse, it may be worth consideration in future trials of catheter ablation within athletic cohorts. Notably, however, a significant improvement in atrial function, determined by speckle-tracking echocardiography, in the 12 months following early ablative treatment has been observed. Those managed without catheter ablation had a progressive worsening of atrial function over the same time period.[68]

Overall, catheter ablation seems to yield similar success rates for athletes compared with nonathletes in the absence of other significant factors such as structural heart disease. However, the data to date have been for a limited number of patients and with modest follow-up. Indeed, emerging data have pointed to the importance of also treating the primary insult in improving the outcomes after ablation.[12,13] Nevertheless, based on current evidence, catheter ablation may be considered an effective treatment option, although current data are limited by small sample sizes and the absence of prospective randomized controlled trials.

Anticoagulation

Given the numerous health benefits of chronic exercise training, athletes typically present with a CHA_2DS_2-VASc less than or equal to 1 and, subsequently, a low risk of systemic thromboembolism.

As such, anticoagulation is seldom necessary in this cohort. A small minority of athletes with a CHA_2DS_2-VASC score greater than or equal to 2, such as female masters athletes older than 65 years or those with hypertension as a comorbidity, may require anticoagulation per recommended guidelines.[56] In such a scenario, it may be necessary to consider the bleeding risk in the setting of contact sports or activities in which there is a higher risk of falls, such as in mountain biking or skiing. Anticoagulation needs to be considered in the older athlete.

FUTURE DIRECTIONS

There remains a distinct absence of prospective, long-term data regarding the effects of exercise training on the heart and the risk of arrhythmias. Future studies that address the potential mechanisms, such as atrial remodeling and autonomic alterations, underlying AF-risk in human athletes will provide significant advancement to the field. This will be difficult given the logistical and financial implications of long-term prospective trials within a large population, yet necessary given the recent surge in endurance sports participation, such as in marathons and long-distance triathlons. Importantly, novel structural and functional cardiac imaging approaches alongside invasive and/or noninvasive electrophysiological mapping techniques are now available to provide a unique insight into the cardiac adaptations that accompany exercise training. Such advances will enable the evaluation of the mechanisms contributing to heightened AF risk in the athletic population. Furthermore, studies that address the treatment options for athletes with arrhythmias will provide the necessary evidence to support decision-making regarding the management of AF in this cohort.

SUMMARY

Extensive endurance training increases the risk of AF mostly due to atrial remodeling, including dilation and fibrosis, alongside autonomic alterations favoring vagal tone and a possible increase in the frequency of atrial ectopic triggers (see

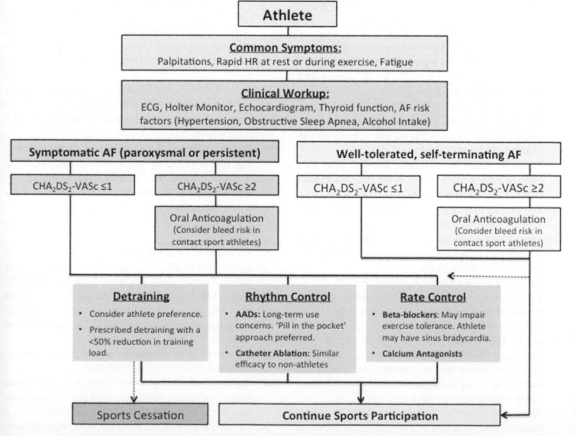

Fig. 2. A schema for the evaluation and treatment of AF in athletes. ECG, electrocardiogram; HR, heart rate.

Fig. 1). Despite the prevalence of AF being well established in human athletes, the mechanistic insights underlying this observation are primarily based on animal studies. Rhythm control using catheter ablation is increasingly used in this cohort due to the poor tolerability of medical therapy. However, data have been limited to single-center studies. Catheter ablation is shown to be equally effective in athletes with AF compared with non-athletes and can thus be considered for the symptomatic athlete seeking rhythm control and a prompt return to sports participation (**Fig. 2**). Prospective studies are warranted to further evaluate the mechanisms promoting AF in human athletes and to evaluate treatment options in this cohort.

REFERENCES

1. Wen CP, Wai JPM, Tsai MK, et al. Minimum amount of physical activity for reduced mortality and extended life expectancy: a prospective cohort study. Lancet 2011;378:1244–53.
2. Lee D-C, Sui X, Artero EG, et al. Long-term effects of changes in cardiorespiratory fitness and body mass index on all-cause and cardiovascular disease mortality in men: the Aerobics Center Longitudinal Study. Circulation 2011;124:2483–90.
3. Myers J, Prakash M, Froelicher V, et al. Exercise capacity and mortality among men referred for exercise testing. N Engl J Med 2002;346:793–801.
4. Lee D-C, Pate RR, Lavie CJ, et al. Leisure-time running reduces all-cause and cardiovascular mortality risk. J Am Coll Cardiol 2014;64:472–81.
5. Marijon E, Tafflet M, Celermajer DS, et al. Sports-related sudden death in the general population. Circulation 2011;124:672–81.
6. Marijon E, Tafflet M, Antero-Jacquemin J, et al. Mortality of French participants in the Tour de France (1947-2012). Eur Heart J 2013;34:3145–50.
7. Heidbüchel H, Hoogsteen J, Fagard R, et al. High prevalence of right ventricular involvement in endurance athletes with ventricular arrhythmias. Role of an electrophysiologic study in risk stratification. Eur Heart J 2003;24:1473–80.
8. Chugh SS, Havmoeller R, Narayanan K, et al. Worldwide epidemiology of atrial fibrillation: a global burden of disease 2010 study. Circulation 2014;129: 837–47.
9. Wong CX, Brooks AG, Leong DP, et al. The increasing burden of atrial fibrillation compared with heart failure and myocardial infarction: a 15-year study of all hospitalizations in Australia. Arch Intern Med 2012;172:739–41.
10. Wong CX, Lau DH, Sanders P. Atrial fibrillation epidemic and hospitalizations: how to turn the rising tide? Circulation 2014;129:2361–3.
11. Patel NJ, Deshmukh A, Pant S, et al. Contemporary trends of hospitalization for atrial fibrillation in the United States, 2000 through 2010: implications for healthcare planning. Circulation 2014;129:2371–9.
12. Pathak RK, Middeldorp ME, Lau DH, et al. Aggressive risk factor reduction study for atrial fibrillation and implications for the outcome of ablation: the arrest-AF cohort study. J Am Coll Cardiol 2014;64: 2222–31.
13. Pathak RK, Middeldorp ME, Meredith M, et al. Long-Term Effect of Goal-Directed Weight Management in an Atrial Fibrillation Cohort: a Long-Term Follow-Up Study (LEGACY study). J Am Coll Cardiol 2015;65: 2159–69.
14. Pathak RK, Elliott A, Middeldorp ME, et al. Impact of CARDIOrespiratory FITness on arrhythmia recurrence in obese individuals with atrial fibrillation: the CARDIO-FIT Study. J Am Coll Cardiol 2015;66:985–96.
15. Karjalainen J, Kujala UM, Kaprio J, et al. Lone atrial fibrillation in vigorously exercising middle aged men: case-control study. BMJ 1998;316:1784–5.
16. Mont L, Sambola A, Brugada J, et al. Long-lasting sport practice and lone atrial fibrillation. Eur Heart J 2002;23:477–82.
17. Elosua R, Arquer A, Mont L, et al. Sport practice and the risk of lone atrial fibrillation: a case-control study. Int J Cardiol 2006;108:332–7.
18. Calvo N, Ramos P, Montserrat S, et al. Emerging risk factors and the dose-response relationship between physical activity and lone atrial fibrillation: a prospective case-control study. Europace 2015;18(1): 57–63.
19. Molina L, Mont L, Marrugat J, et al. Long-term endurance sport practice increases the incidence of lone atrial fibrillation in men: a follow-up study. Europace 2008;10:618–23.
20. Wilhelm M, Roten L, Tanner H, et al. Atrial remodeling, autonomic tone, and lifetime training hours in nonelite athletes. Am J Cardiol 2011;108:580–5.
21. Baldesberger S, Bauersfeld U, Candinas R, et al. Sinus node disease and arrhythmias in the long-term follow-up of former professional cyclists. Eur Heart J 2008;29:71–8.
22. Andersen K, Farahmand B, Ahlbom A, et al. Risk of arrhythmias in 52 755 long-distance cross-country skiers: a cohort study. Eur Heart J 2013;34:3624–31.
23. Myrstad M, Nystad W, Graff-Iversen S, et al. Effect of years of endurance exercise on risk of atrial fibrillation and atrial flutter. Am J Cardiol 2014;114: 1229–33.
24. Wilhelm M. Atrial fibrillation in endurance athletes. Eur J Prev Cardiol 2013;21:1040–8.
25. Nattel S, Harada M. Atrial remodeling and atrial fibrillation: recent advances and translational perspectives. J Am Coll Cardiol 2014;63:2335–45.
26. Lau DH, Mackenzie L, Kelly DJ, et al. Hypertension and atrial fibrillation: evidence of progressive atrial

remodeling with electrostructural correlate in a conscious chronically instrumented ovine model. Heart Rhythm 2010;7:1282–90.

27. Dimitri H, Ng M, Brooks AG, et al. Atrial remodeling in obstructive sleep apnea: implications for atrial fibrillation. Heart Rhythm 2012;9:321–7.

28. Mahajan R, Lau DH, Brooks AG, et al. Electrophysiological, electroanatomical, and structural remodeling of the atria as consequences of sustained obesity. J Am Coll Cardiol 2015;66:1–11.

29. Baggish AL. Mechanisms underlying the cardiac benefits of exercise: still running in the dark. Trends Cardiovasc Med 2015;25:537–9.

30. Pelliccia A, Maron BJ, Di Paolo FM, et al. Prevalence and clinical significance of left atrial remodeling in competitive athletes. J Am Coll Cardiol 2005;46: 690–6.

31. Mont L, Tamborero D, Elosua R, et al. Physical activity, height, and left atrial size are independent risk factors for lone atrial fibrillation in middle-aged healthy individuals. Europace 2008;10:15–20.

32. Wilson M, O'Hanlon R, Basavarajaiah S, et al. Cardiovascular function and the veteran athlete. Eur J Appl Physiol 2010;110:459–78.

33. La Gerche A, Burns AT, D'Hooge J, et al. Exercise strain rate imaging demonstrates normal right ventricular contractile reserve and clarifies ambiguous resting measures in endurance athletes. J Am Soc Echocardiogr 2012;25:253–62.e1.

34. Guasch E, Benito B, Qi X, et al. Atrial fibrillation promotion by endurance exercise: demonstration and mechanistic exploration in an animal model. J Am Coll Cardiol 2013;62:68–77.

35. Benito B, Gay-Jordi G, Serrano-Mollar A, et al. Cardiac arrhythmogenic remodeling in a rat model of long-term intensive exercise training. Circulation 2011;123:13–22.

36. Schotten U, Verheule S, Kirchhof P, et al. Pathophysiological mechanisms of atrial fibrillation: a translational appraisal. Physiol Rev 2011;91:265–325.

37. La Gerche A, Inder WJ, Roberts TJ, et al. Relationship between inflammatory cytokines and indices of cardiac dysfunction following intense endurance exercise. PLoS One 2015;10:e0130031.

38. Sugama K, Suzuki K, Yoshitani K, et al. Changes of thioredoxin, oxidative stress markers, inflammation and muscle/renal damage following intensive endurance exercise. Exerc Immunol Rev 2015;21: 130–42.

39. Aschar-Sobbi R, Izaddoustdar F, Korogyi AS, et al. Increased atrial arrhythmia susceptibility induced by intense endurance exercise in mice requires TNFα. Nat Commun 2015;6:6018.

40. Sun M, Chen M, Dawood F, et al. Tumor necrosis factor-alpha mediates cardiac remodeling and ventricular dysfunction after pressure overload state. Circulation 2007;115:1398–407.

41. Luepker RV, Holmberg S, Varnauskas E. Left atrial pressure during exercise in hemodynamic normals. Am Heart J 1971;81:494–7.

42. Reeves JT, Groves BM, Cymerman A, et al. Operation Everest II: cardiac filling pressures during cycle exercise at sea level. Respir Physiol 1990;80:147–54.

43. Aubert AE, Seps B, Beckers F. Heart rate variability in athletes. Sports Med 2003;33:889–919.

44. Takahashi Y, Jaïs P, Hocini M, et al. Shortening of fibrillatory cycle length in the pulmonary vein during vagal excitation. J Am Coll Cardiol 2006;47:774–80.

45. Coumel P. Paroxysmal atrial fibrillation: a disorder of autonomic tone? Eur Heart J 1994;15(Suppl A):9–16.

46. Bettoni M, Zimmermann M. Autonomic tone variations before the onset of paroxysmal atrial fibrillation. Circulation 2002;105:2753–9.

47. Haïssaguerre M, Jaïs P, Shah DC, et al. Spontaneous initiation of atrial fibrillation by ectopic beats originating in the pulmonary veins. N Engl J Med 1998;339:659–66.

48. Brooks AG, Rangnekar G, Ganesan AN, et al. Characteristics of ectopic triggers associated with paroxysmal and persistent atrial fibrillation: evidence for a changing role. Heart Rhythm 2012;9:1367–74.

49. Zipes DP, Link MS, Ackerman MJ, et al. Eligibility and Disqualification Recommendations for Competitive Athletes With Cardiovascular Abnormalities: Task Force 9: Arrhythmias and Conduction Defects: a Scientific Statement from the American Heart Association and American College of Cardiology. J Am Coll Cardiol 2015;66(21): 2412–23.

50. Furlanello F, Bertoldi A, Dallago M, et al. Atrial fibrillation in elite athletes. J Cardiovasc Electrophysiol 1998;9:S63–8.

51. Weiner RB, Wang F, Berkstresser B, et al. Regression of "gray zone" exercise-induced concentric left ventricular hypertrophy during prescribed detraining. J Am Coll Cardiol 2012;59:1992–4.

52. Pelliccia A. Remodeling of left ventricular hypertrophy in elite athletes after long-term deconditioning. Circulation 2002;105:944–9.

53. Stein R, Medeiros CM, Rosito GA, et al. Intrinsic sinus and atrioventricular node electrophysiologic adaptations in endurance athletes. J Am Coll Cardiol 2002;39:1033–8.

54. D'Souza A, Bucchi A, Johnsen AB, et al. Exercise training reduces resting heart rate via downregulation of the funny channel HCN4. Nat Commun 2014;5:3775.

55. Brosnan M, La Gerche A, Kumar S, et al. Modest agreement in ECG interpretation limits the application of ECG screening in young athletes. Heart Rhythm 2015;12:130–6.

56. January CT, Wann LS, Alpert JS, et al. 2014 AHA/ACC/HRS Guideline for the Management of Patients with Atrial Fibrillation: Executive Summary: A Report

of the American College of Cardiology/American Heart Association Task Force on Practice Guidelines and the Heart Rhythm Society. Circulation 2014; 130(23):2071–104.

57. Joyner MJ, Freund BJ, Jilka SM, et al. Effects of beta-blockade on exercise capacity of trained and untrained men: a hemodynamic comparison. J Appl Physiol (1985) 1986;60:1429–34.

58. Jilka SM, Joyner MJ, Nittolo JM, et al. Maximal exercise responses to acute and chronic beta-adrenergic blockade in healthy male subjects. Med Sci Sports Exerc 1988;20:570–3.

59. Kindermann W. Calcium antagonists and exercise performance. Sports Med 1987;4:177–93.

60. Alboni P, Botto GL, Baldi N, et al. Outpatient treatment of recent-onset atrial fibrillation with the "pill-in-the-pocket" approach. N Engl J Med 2004; 351:2384–91.

61. Taylor R, Gandhi MM, Lloyd G. Tachycardia due to atrial flutter with rapid 1:1 conduction following treatment of atrial fibrillation with flecainide. BMJ 2010;340:b4684.

62. Gupta A, Perera T, Ganesan A, et al. Complications of catheter ablation of atrial fibrillation: a systematic review. Circ Arrhythm Electrophysiol 2013;6:1082–8.

63. Furlanello F, Lupo P, Pittalis M, et al. Radiofrequency catheter ablation of atrial fibrillation in athletes referred for disabling symptoms preventing usual training schedule and sport competition. J Cardiovasc Electrophysiol 2008;19:457–62.

64. Calvo N, Mont L, Tamborero D, et al. Efficacy of circumferential pulmonary vein ablation of atrial fibrillation in endurance athletes. Europace 2010; 12:30–6.

65. Koopman P, Nuyens D, Garweg C, et al. Efficacy of radiofrequency catheter ablation in athletes with atrial fibrillation. Europace 2011;13:1386–93.

66. Mugnai G, de Asmundis C, Ciconte G, et al. Incidence and characteristics of complications in the setting of second-generation cryoballoon ablation: a large single-center study of 500 consecutive patients. Heart Rhythm 2015;12:1476–82.

67. Wong GR, Lau DH, Baillie TJ, et al. Novel use of sildenafil in the management of pulmonary hypertension due to post-catheter ablation 'stiff left atrial syndrome'. Int J Cardiol 2015;181:55–6.

68. Walters TE, Nisbet A, Morris GM, et al. Progression of atrial remodeling in patients with high burden atrial fibrillation: implications for early ablative intervention. Heart Rhythm 2016;13(2):331–9.

Congenital Heart Disease and the Athlete
What We Know and What We Do Not Know

 CrossMark

Peter N. Dean, MD[a],*, Robert W. Battle, MD[a,b]

KEYWORDS

- Congenital heart disease • Sports participation • Exercise • Quality of life • Sudden cardiac arrest

KEY POINTS

- Athletes with congenital heart disease (CHD) will pose a dilemma for practitioners.
- There are no randomized trials evaluating competitive athletic participation versus restriction in athletes with CHD.
- There is evidence supporting sports participation as beneficial to individuals.
- There are no data that demonstrate that withdrawal from sports in CHD saves lives.
- Although practitioners should consult the guidelines, they should also be aware of the overall lack of evidence supporting restriction and they should individualize recommendations for each patient, including involving patients and families in shared decision-making and risk assessment.

CASE EXAMPLES

A 20-year-old college cyclist born with critical pulmonary stenosis underwent balloon valvuloplasty as a neonate. Because of severe pulmonary valve insufficiency, at 15 years of age he underwent pulmonary valve repair and was left with residual severe pulmonary valve insufficiency. He now has a significantly increased right ventricular end diastolic volume of 177 mL/m^2 with an ejection fraction of 41% by cardiac MRI after his first year in college when he increased his training regimen dramatically. His cardiopulmonary exercise stress test demonstrates a maximum oxygen consumption of 46.4 mL/kg/min (96% predicted).[1] He is one of the stronger climbers on his college team. Should he continue competing?

A 22-year-old woman was born with pulmonary atresia with an intact ventricular septum (single

ventricle physiology); she has had a lateral tunnel Fontan procedure and is asymptomatic (without history of syncope, arrhythmias, or thromboembolic complications) and has had normal ventricular systolic function on echocardiogram, normal Holter monitors, and normal oxygen saturations. She has been competing in triathalons, during which she can run a mile in less than 9 minutes and swim a mile in less than 30 minutes. Should she continue competing?

An 18-year-old male collegiate lacrosse player was found to have a bicuspid aortic valve (right, non–cusp fusion), moderate aortic valve insufficiency, no aortic valve stenosis, and mildly dilated aortic root. His echocardiogram measurements showed a left ventricular internal diameter of 6.2 mm with normal systolic function, an aortic root diameter of 4.0 cm, and an ascending aorta diameter of 3.3 cm.[2] Should he be allowed to participate?

Disclosure Statement: The authors have nothing to disclose.
[a] Division of Pediatric Cardiology, Department of Pediatrics, University of Virginia, 1204 West Main Street, Charlottesville, VA 22908, USA; [b] Division of Cardiology, Department of Internal Medicine, University of Virginia, 1204 West Main Street, Charlottesville, VA 22908, USA
* Corresponding author. Department of Pediatrics, University of Virginia, PO Box 800386, 1204 West Main Street, Charlottesville, VA 22908.
E-mail address: pnd8j@virginia.edu

Cardiol Clin 34 (2016) 579–589
http://dx.doi.org/10.1016/j.ccl.2016.06.007
0733-8651/16/© 2016 Elsevier Inc. All rights reserved.

INTRODUCTION

Since outcomes for patients with congenital heart disease (CHD) have greatly improved, most patients with CHD are surviving into adulthood and seeking high-quality lives. Many patients with CHD, even those with the most severe CHD, will have normal or near normal exercise capacity.[3–5] Because these patients are doing better and feeling better, they are creating dilemmas for practitioners in regard to competitive sports participation. The risk of sudden cardiac arrest (SCA) is balanced by the well-known benefits of habitual exercise; therefore, these dilemmas and decisions are very complex with important consequences to athletes.

Much of the conversation and literature in the sports cardiology field has focused on patients with no known heart disease.[6–8] There is less evidence for patients with known heart disease, specifically CHD. Much time, effort, and expertise has gone into developing the new American Heart Association (AHA)/American College of Cardiology's (ACC) guidelines and the European Society of Cardiology's guidelines; but these are primarily based on expert opinion and not a solid foundation of scientific evidence (**Tables 1–3**).[9–15] Given the possible complexity of CHD and differences in individual physiology and surgical repair, it is also unlikely that any guideline or consensus document will ever be able to completely address every individual patient. Furthermore, these guidelines only address competitive sports participation and not recreational sports participation.

The goal of this article is to review the literature regarding competitive sports participation in patients with CHD and to acknowledge where the evidence is lacking to support those recommendations.

THE CASE FOR PARTICIPATION

These dilemmas are often brought to physicians' attention because of the perceived benefits of sports participation to patients and families. There is considerable evidence supporting sports participation as beneficial to individuals.

First, in healthy populations, sports participation seems to be important for children's self-esteem and social inclusion and may improve academic performance.[16–18]

Second, sports participation is a method for children to engage in aerobic exercise and physical activity, which has been recommended[19] and has been shown to benefit patients with CHD.[20–24] Increased leisure-time physical activity has also been shown to correlate with better endothelial function in healthy patients,[25] which is something that will be important for the long-term health of patients with CHD.

Third, competitive sports participation specifically in individuals with CHD seems to be have health benefits. Sports participation has been shown to correlate with improved quality-of-life scores, improved exercise capacity, and lower body mass indexes.[26,27] Sports participation has also been associated with lower neurohormone levels and increased event-free survival.[28]

Lastly, there have been studies looking at sports participation in other cardiac diseases (long QT syndrome[29] and patients with implantable cardioverter-defibrillators[30–32]) that have shown that participation can be safely achieved.

RESTRICTING PATIENTS SHOULD NOT BE TAKEN LIGHTLY (AND ONLY DONE WHEN THERE IS EVIDENCE TO RESTRICT AND NOT THE OTHER WAY AROUND)

Although restricting patients may be an easy decision when there is controversy or a lack of data, restricting patients is far from a benign recommendation.

First, preventing an athlete from participation has profound quality-of-life and psychological consequences.[26,33] For many adolescents and young adults, playing a sport and being on a team provides them with a social structure and gives them a strong sense of identity.

Second, restricting athletes may also provide a false sense of security. A study of patients who were restricted because of an inherited arrhythmia syndrome found patients still spent significant time performing unsupervised vigorous to very vigorous activities during routine daily living.[34] Not only can we never fully restrict a patient from activities of daily living but these patients also have a risk of sudden death even if they are not participating in competitive physical activity. A recent international study also showed that only 10% of sudden deaths in adults with CHD were associated with exercise, with the majority occurring during rest (69%) or sleep (11%).[35]

Lastly, restricting patients will also increase the risk of obesity, which is a well-recognized problem in patients with CHD[36–38] and has significant consequences if our goal is for patients to age well with a normal life expectancy.

THE CASE FOR RESTRICTION

The most compelling argument for sports restriction in any disease is to prevent SCA that otherwise might not have occurred. Obviously, this is

Table 1
American Heart Association/American College of Cardiology's recommendations and level of evidence for shunt lesions

Cardiac Anatomy	Recommendations	Class	Level of Evidence
Small ASD with normal RV and no pulmonary hypertension	Full participation	I	C
Large ASD and no pulmonary hypertension	Full participation	I	C
ASD and pulmonary hypertension	Allowed to participate in IA sports	I	C
ASD and pulmonary vascular disease, cyanosis, and right to left shunt	Restricted from all competitive sports, with the possible exception of IA	III	C
History of ASD repair or device and no pulmonary hypertension	Full participation	I	C
History of ASD repair or device and residual pulmonary hypertension, arrhythmias, or myocardial dysfunction	Allowed to participate in IA sports	IIb	C
Small or restrictive VSD with normal RV size and no pulmonary hypertension	Full participation	I	C
Large, hemodynamically significant VSD and pulmonary hypertension	Allowed to participate in IA sports	IIb	C
History of VSD repair with no pulmonary hypertension, arrhythmias, or myocardial dysfunction	Full participation	I	C
History of VSD repair and residual pulmonary hypertension	Allowed to participate in IA sports	I	B
History of VSD repair with mild to moderate pulmonary hypertension or ventricular dysfunction	Restricted from all competitive sports, with the possible exception of IA	III	C
Small PDA with normal pulmonary artery pressures and normal left heart chambers	Full participation	I	C
Moderate to large PDA with persistent pulmonary hypertension	Only allowed to participate in IA sports	I	B
Moderate to large PDA with left ventricular enlargement	Full restrictions	III	C
History of surgical or catheter PDA closure and no evidence of pulmonary hypertension	Full participation	I	C
History of surgical or catheter PDA closure and residual pulmonary hypertension	Restricted from all competitive sports, with the possible exception of IA	I	B

Abbreviations: ASD, atrial septal defect; PDA, patent ductus arteriosus; RV, right ventricle; VSD, ventricular septal defect.

From Van Hare GF, Ackerman MJ, Evangelista JA, et al. Eligibility and disqualification recommendations for competitive athletes with cardiovascular abnormalities: task force 4: congenital heart disease: a scientific statement from the American Heart Association and American College of Cardiology. J Am Coll Cardiol 2015;66(21):2372–84; with permission.

Table 2
American Heart Association/American College of Cardiology's recommendations and level of evidence for obstructed/valvular lesions

Cardiac Anatomy	Recommendations	Class	Level of Evidence
Mild pulmonary valve stenosis and normal RV function	Full participation	I	B
Moderate or severe pulmonary valve stenosis	Allowed to participate in IA and IB sports	IIb	B
History of pulmonary valve surgery or balloon valvuloplasty and gradient <40 mm Hg	Full participation	I	B
Severe pulmonary insufficiency with marked RV enlargement	Allowed to participate in IA and IB sports	IIb	B
Mild aortic valve stenosis	Full participation	I	B
Moderate aortic valve stenosis	Allowed to participate in IA, IB, IIA sports	IIb	B
Severe aortic valve stenosis	Allowed to participate in IA sports	I	B
Severe aortic valve stenosis	Restricted from all competitive sports, with the possible exception of IA	III	B
Residual aortic valve stenosis after surgical or catheter intervention	Considered for participation based on untreated recommendations	IIb	C
Untreated coarctation of the aorta without ascending aorta dilation and normal exercise test and <20 mm Hg blood pressure gradient	Full participation	I	C
Untreated coarctation of the aorta and blood pressure gradient >20 mm Hg or abnormal exercise stress test or significant ascending aorta dilation	Allowed to participate in IA sports	IIb	C
History of coarctation repair or stent and blood pressure gradient <20 mm Hg, normal exercise test, no ascending aorta dilation, no aneurysm, and no concomitant aortic valve disease	Allowed to participate in IA, IB, IC, I A, IIB, IIC sports	IIb	C
History of coarctation of the aorta repair or stent and significant aortic dilation or aneurysm	Allowed to participate in IA and IB sports	IIb	C

Abbreviation: RV, right ventricle.

From Van Hare GF, Ackerman MJ, Evangelista JA, et al. Eligibility and disqualification recommendations for competitive athletes with cardiovascular abnormalities: task force 4: congenital heart disease: a scientific statement From the American Heart Association and American College of Cardiology. J Am Coll Cardiol 2015;66(21):2372–84; with permission.

Table 3
American Heart Association/American College of Cardiology's recommendations and level of evidence for cyanotic or palliated congenital heart disease

Cardiac Anatomy	Recommendations	Class	Level of Evidence
Unrepaired cyanotic heart disease who are clinically stable and asymptomatic	Allowed to participate in IA sports	IIb	C
History of TOF repair and no ventricular dysfunction, arrhythmias, or outflow tract obstruction and a normal exercise test	Full participation	IIb	B
History of TOF repair and severe ventricular dysfunction, severe outflow tract obstruction or recurrent or uncontrolled atrial or ventricular arrhythmias	Restricted from all competitive sports, with the possible exception of IA	III	B
History of Mustard or Senning procedure operation for d-TGA arteries if they have no arrhythmias or ventricular dysfunction	Allowed to participate in IA, IB, IIA, IIB sports	IIb	C
History of Mustard or Senning procedure operation for d-TGA and a history of arrhythmias, RV dysfunction, or severe RV outflow tract obstruction	Restricted from all competitive sports, with the possible exception of IA	III	C
CCTGA without arrhythmias, ventricular dysfunction, exercise intolerance, or exercise-induced ischemia	Participation in IA and IB sports and may be considered for IIA, IIB, IIIB and IIIB	IIb	C
CCTGA severe clinical systemic RV dysfunction, severe RV outflow tract dysfunction, or recurrent or uncontrolled atrial or ventricular arrhythmias	Restricted from all competitive sports, with the possible exception of IA	III	C
History of arterial switch procedure for d-TGA without symptoms, normal ventricular function and no tachyarrhythmias	Full participation	IIb	C
History of arterial switch procedure for d-TGA and more than mild hemodynamic abnormalities or ventricular dysfunction with normal exercise testing	Allowed to participate in IA, IB, IC and IIA	IIb	C
History of arterial switch procedure for d-TGA with evidence of ischemia	Restricted from all sports with possible exception of IA	III	B
History of Fontan procedure with no symptoms and no hemodynamic abnormalities	Allowed to participate in IA sports	I	C
History of Fontan procedure without evidence of abnormalities on exercise stress test	Sports may be considered on individual basis	IIb	C
Mild to moderate Ebstein anomaly without cyanosis, normal RV size, less than moderate tricuspid valve regurgitation, and no arrhythmias	Full participation	IIb	C
Ebstein anomaly with severe tricuspid valve regurgitation but no arrhythmias	Allowed to participate in IA sports	IIb	C

Abbreviations: CCTGA, congenitally corrected transposition of the great arteries; RV, right ventricle; TGA, transposition of the great arteries; TOF, tetralogy of Fallot.
From Van Hare GF, Ackerman MJ, Evangelista JA, et al. Eligibility and disqualification recommendations for competitive athletes with cardiovascular abnormalities: task force 4: congenital heart disease: a scientific statement from the American Heart Association and American College of Cardiology. J Am Coll Cardiol 2015;66(21):2372–84; with permission.

a catastrophic event and one that should be avoided if possible. The first Bethesda guideline[39] acknowledged the absence of data to support sports restriction as a way to prevent SCA, and this is largely true today. Another argument for restriction is the possibility that stressing the heart or exercise will worsen the natural history of the disease (ie, speed progression of heart failure or create arrhythmias).

Although there may be controversies for sports participation in some diseases, there are some in which restriction is not controversial and should be universal. Diseases such as the Marfan syndrome with a significantly dilated aortic root, severe aortic valve stenosis, symptomatic patients with anomalous coronary artery origins, or catecholaminergic polymorphic ventricular tachycardia have evidence and solid rationale for sports restriction.[9] There are also sports and diseases that should not be paired and require restrictions (eg, football or boxing in a patient on anticoagulation therapy, power lifting in a patients with Marfan syndrome or another aortopathy, high-altitude hiking in a patient with pulmonary hypertension, or activities in patients who are pacemaker dependent because of the risk for lead damage).

WHAT IS KNOWN ABOUT THE SUBJECT
Risk of Sudden Death in Patients with Congenital Heart Disease

We know there is risk of sudden cardiac death in patients with CHD[40,41] and that some lesions are higher risk than others. It seems that the lesions that are at highest risk for SCA (irrespective of exercise) are patients with systemic right ventricles, left ventricular outflow tract lesions, tetralogy of Fallot, and Eisenmenger syndrome.[35,42,43] We also know that the risk of SCA is related to exercise in only the minority of cases. Only 10% of sudden deaths in adults with CHD were associated with exercise. The rest of the sudden deaths occurred during rest (69%) or sleep (11%).[35] Sports participation was also shown to not be associated with adverse cardiac events in a Dutch population with a variety of types of CHD.[27]

Physiologic Changes with Exercise

In general, in order to provide oxygen to the working muscle the heart increases cardiac output by increasing the heart rate and increasing stroke volume.[44] The interactions between the muscles, lungs, and heart determine the capacity of the heart to increase the cardiac output and will be different for patients with CHD. For example, because patients with single ventricle physiology

who have had a Fontan procedure do not have a subpulmonary pump, the ability of the heart to increase cardiac output will depend on pulmonary vascular resistance and ventricular relaxation, which allows for increased preload and increased stroke volume.[45,46] Exercise can also effect the systolic blood pressure, with isometric exercises causing a large increase in systolic blood pressures (which may have significant implications for patients with aortic aneurysms or the Marfan syndrome) and isotonic exercises having a less effect on systolic blood pressure.[47,48]

Chronically, these hemodynamic changes needed to increase cardiac output create either a pressure load or a volume load on the heart. These loads will cause cardiac adaptations over time depending on the type, duration, and intensity of training.[49-52] These chronic adaptations can be compounded when combined with CHD and can potentially amplify chamber dilation and hypertrophy.[1]

Exercise Training and Sports Improve Short-term Fitness Measurements

As reviewed in 2 recent review articles on the subject,[53,54] there are data addressing the effectiveness and safety of exercise programs for children with CHD. Duppen and colleagues[53] showed that the risk of adverse events was very low (4 out of 621 patients, and none seem to be directly related to exercise program) and there were no cases of SCA with exercise programs in any of the articles. Although there was a wide range of exercise program designs, most studies demonstrated a positive effect on the cardiac health (as measured by B-type natriuretic peptide, cardiac MRI, and electrocardiogram) and a positive effect on overall exercise capacity (measured by oxygen consumption and 6-minute walk test). These positive effects of the training program also seem to persist in the medium term (4–10 months after stopping the training program).[20,55,56]

Not just exercise but sports participation in itself also seems to correlate with improved quality-of-life scores, improved exercise capacity and lower body mass indexes.[26,27] Sports participation was also associated with lower neurohormone levels and increased event-free survival.[28]

Physicians Do Not Universally Follow the Congenital Heart Disease Sports Participation Guidelines

Nationwide the guidelines are not universally followed,[26,57-59] and this suggests that patients and physicians think that participation outweighs the risk. Although guidelines are helpful, there is still room for physicians to deviate from the guidelines when there is good reason, a thoughtful discussion with the patients and families, and allowance for some assumed risk to be accepted by the athlete and family.[38,60,61]

If Sudden Cardiac Arrest Occurs, the Athlete May Be Safer at a Training Facility or Sporting Event Instead of an Unsupervised Setting

If a cardiac arrest does occur, several studies have demonstrated that survival is better if a cardiac arrest occurs in public compared with home[62,63]; certain public settings (casinos[64] and airplanes[65]) have also demonstrated the importance of a quick response and use of automatic external defibrillators. Recently Marijon and colleagues[66] also demonstrated that survival after sports-related cardiac arrest events was better if the event occurred at a sports facility compared with an event outside of a sports facility.

WHAT IS NOT KNOWN ABOUT THE SUBJECT
The Risk of Sudden Death with Exercise in Each Patient with Congenital Heart Disease

There are no randomized trials evaluating competitive athletic participation versus restriction in athletes with CHD. Existing studies are case series, retrospective population studies, and registries. There are no data that demonstrate that withdrawal from sports in CHD saves lives.

The authors do not have a consistent strategy to risk stratify patients with CHD who are at risk for sudden death with exercise.[67] In the previously cited articles regarding sudden death (at anytime, not just with exercise) in patients with CHD,[35,42,43] the authors have identified higher-risk patients (systemic right ventricles, left ventricular outflow tract lesions, tetralogy of Fallot, and Eisenmenger syndrome); but there are still patients who die suddenly with other types of CHD, and there are patients who have these lesions but have not had any events. Even if one were to just look at the high-risk lesions, the anatomy and physiology is different for each one, so it is unlikely that there is a uniform cause of SCA for the group.

Long-term Physiologic Changes Due to Exercise

Although we may understand the acute and chronic cardiac changes with exercise and the improvement with exercise training programs, we do not fully understand those changes and how they interact with the heart with congenital disease. Would chronic adaptations related to habitual exercise alter the natural history or course

for patients with CHD? Does exercise improve the hemodynamics and improve the long-term survival for patients with single ventricle physiology? For patients with tetralogy of Fallot and pulmonary valve insufficiency, does chronic exercise improve their right ventricular function or does it promote dilation and worsen right ventricular function? Does exercise have any role in worsening aortic root dilation in patients with Marfan syndrome, bicuspid aortic valve, or CHD? Do patients with single ventricle and Fontan physiology have less heart failure symptoms or less thromboembolic complications if they are physically active?

Can You Positively Motivate Somebody to Participate in Sports or to Exercise?

Motivating patients to change their behaviors (lose weight, exercise, stop smoking, and so forth) is very complex and often not successful. It is difficult for a physician to motivate a sedentary adult patient to begin participating in a sport or start an exercise program. The window of opportunity may be early in patients' lives, when we can reassure families that their infant or young child should be able to participate in sports and exercise and guiding the family toward recommended activities. Because many parents are inappropriately afraid of SCA in their child with CHD[68] and one of the reasons for lack of participation is lack of self-efficacy,[69] early encouragement and reassurance when appropriate would likely benefit most patients with CHD.

RETURNING TO THE CASE EXAMPLES

The example of the 22-year-old cyclist is a good example of the interplay between CHD and the cardiac effects of endurance training. With his strong endurance training history, the right ventricular enlargement is likely due to a combination of volume loading from both the pulmonary valve insufficiency and endurance training. This point is demonstrated by the fact that when he detrained his right ventricular end diastolic volume decreased to 155 mL/m^2.[1] Given the anatomy and elite training it is difficulty to fit the AHA/ACC's guidelines to this patient perfectly. If one were to be rigid about the guidelines, he would likely be restricted to 1A and 1B sports because the recommendation reads, "athletes with severe pulmonary insufficiency as demonstrated by marked RV enlargement can consider participation in low-intensity class IA and IB sports."[10] The authors think the evidence is lacking to support this recommendation, and the exercise capacity of this athlete would support a favorable physiology over an unfavorable one.

The 22-year-old triathlete with pulmonary atresia who has had a Fontan procedure is a good example of a patient with complex physiology whereby the cardiologist will need to weigh risks versus benefits of exercise in an area with little amount of evidence to guide us. According to the AHA/ACC's guidelines, she would be restricted from participation because triathlons are considered a high-static and high-dynamic (3C) sport.[70] The AHA/ACC's recent guidelines recommend only participation in low-static and low dynamic (1A) sports.[10] Despite this restriction, the guidelines state that "participation in other sports may be considered on an individual basis with regard for athletes ability to complete an exercise test without exercise induced arrhythmias, hypotension, ischemia and other concerning clinical symptoms."[10] The guidelines then cite articles that describe risk factors for death and mode of death for patients who have had Fontan procedures.[71,72] Those risk factors were heart failure symptoms, arrhythmias, and atriopulmonary connections; the mode of death is usually thromboembolic, sudden or heart failure related. Although the rate of sudden death is concerning in sports cardiology, no patients were described as participating in exercise or sports at the time of the sudden death. The authors think that her endurance training may prevent venous stasis, thus, protect against thromboembolic complications given her Fontan physiology with a direct cavopulmonary anastomosis and no right ventricle. The use of muscles of the arms and legs promote a reduction in venous stasis and improved venous return to the pulmonary arteries.

The 18-year-old male college lacrosse player who has a bicuspid valve and mildly dilated aortic root is a good example of modifying training regimens to provide safer participation instead of complete restriction. The left ventricular dimension of 6.2 cm is likely due to a combination of athletic training superimposed on the volume load of moderate aortic valve regurgitation. The recommendations for an aortic root dilation of 4.0 cm would restrict him to low- and moderate-static sports (he would be allowed to participate in IA, IB, IC, IIA, IIB, and IIC sports) with "low likelihood of significant bodily contact" and "avoidance of intense weight training should be considered."[73] Lacrosse is considered a moderate-static and high-dynamic sport (IIC) with "risk for bodily contact," so he, therefore, would be restricted.[70] Despite this, given the patient's desire to participate and his personal knowledge of the risks, he has been allowed to continue to participate with close surveillance of his aortic valve and aortic root and restriction from intense weight lifting, which can lead to dramatic increases in mean arterial pressure and may increase the risk of aortic dissection.[74] This case is pertinent as this is the most common congenital defect seen and has a high prevalence in elite athletes,[75] most of whom will have some degree of aortic involvement.

SUMMARY

Athletes with CHD will pose a dilemma for practitioners. Although practitioners should consult the guidelines, they should also be aware of the overall lack of evidence supporting restriction and they should individualize recommendations for each patient, including involving patients and families in shared decision-making. Medical practice is rapidly evolving toward shared decision-making and risk assumption between the physician and patients, which becomes even more critical when evidence is lacking to support one recommendation over another. The authors think that the practice of strictly adhering to current guideline recommendations when counseling most patients with CHD is unfair and may also be incorrect in some instances. The authors agree with the more fair approach that is recommended in a recent article by Terri Fried: "Let me tell you about the pros and cons of options x and y so that you can decide which one matches your priorities."[76]

REFERENCES

1. Hoyt WJ Jr, Dean PN, John AS, et al. Endurance training on congenital valvular regurgitation: an athlete case series. Med Sci Sports Exerc 2016; 48(1):16–9.
2. Hoyt W. Bicuspid aortic valve in two brothers and college lacrosse players. Presented at American College of Cardiology 64th Scientific Session. San Diego (CA), March 15, 2015.
3. Muller J, Bohm B, Semsch S, et al. Currently, children with congenital heart disease are not limited in their submaximal exercise performance. Eur J Cardiothorac Surg 2013;43(6):1096–100.
4. Mahle WT, Wernovsky G, Bridges ND, et al. Impact of early ventricular unloading on exercise performance in preadolescents with single ventricle Fontan physiology. J Am Coll Cardiol 1999;34(5):1637–43.
5. Paridon SM, Mitchell PD, Colan SD, et al. A cross-sectional study of exercise performance during the first 2 decades of life after the Fontan operation. J Am Coll Cardiol 2008;52(2):99–107.
6. Maron BJ, Haas TS, Murphy CJ, et al. Incidence and causes of sudden death in U.S. college athletes. J Am Coll Cardiol 2014;63(16):1636–43.
7. Roberts WO, Stovitz SD. Incidence of sudden cardiac death in Minnesota high school athletes 1993-2012

screened with a standardized pre-participation evaluation. J Am Coll Cardiol 2013;62(14):1298–301.

8. Asif IM, Rao AL, Drezner JA. Sudden cardiac death in young athletes: what is the role of screening? Curr Opin Cardiol 2013;28(1):55–62.

9. Maron BJ, Zipes DP, Kovacs RJ. Eligibility and disqualification recommendations for competitive athletes with cardiovascular abnormalities: preamble, principles, and general considerations: a scientific statement from the American Heart Association and American College of Cardiology. J Am Coll Cardiol 2015;66(21):2343–9.

10. Van Hare GF, Ackerman MJ, Evangelista JK, et al. Eligibility and disqualification recommendations for competitive athletes with cardiovascular abnormalities: task force 4: congenital heart disease: a scientific statement from the American Heart Association and American College of Cardiology. J Am Coll Cardiol 2015;66(21):2372–84.

11. Bonow RO, Nishimura RA, Thompson PD, et al. Eligibility and disqualification recommendations for competitive athletes with cardiovascular abnormalities: task force 5: valvular heart disease: a scientific statement from the American Heart Association and American College of Cardiology. J Am Coll Cardiol 2015;66(21):2385–92.

12. Hirth A, Reybrouck T, Bjarnason-Wehrens B, et al. Recommendations for participation in competitive and leisure sports in patients with congenital heart disease: a consensus document. Eur J Cardiovasc Prev Rehabil 2006;13(3):293–9.

13. Pelliccia A, Fagard R, Bjornstad HH, et al. Recommendations for competitive sports participation in athletes with cardiovascular disease: a consensus document from the Study Group of Sports Cardiology of the Working Group of Cardiac Rehabilitation and Exercise Physiology and the Working Group of Myocardial and Pericardial Diseases of the European Society of Cardiology. Eur Heart J 2005;26(14): 1422–45.

14. Pelliccia A, Zipes DP, Maron BJ. Bethesda conference #36 and the European Society of Cardiology consensus recommendations revisited: a comparison of U.S. and European criteria for eligibility and disqualification of competitive athletes with cardiovascular abnormalities. J Am Coll Cardiol 2008; 52(24):1990–6.

15. Moola F, McCrindle BW, Longmuir PE. Physical activity participation in youth with surgically corrected congenital heart disease: devising guidelines so Johnny can participate. Paediatr Child Health 2009; 14(3):167–70.

16. Dishman RK, Hales DP, Pfeiffer KA, et al. Physical self-concept and self-esteem mediate cross-sectional relations of physical activity and sport participation with depression symptoms among adolescent girls. Health Psychol 2006;25(3):396–407.

17. Babiss LA, Gangwisch JE. Sports participation as a protective factor against depression and suicidal ideation in adolescents as mediated by self-esteem and social support. J Dev Behav Pediatr 2009;30(5): 376–84.

18. Fox CK, Barr-Anderson D, Neumark-Sztainer D, et al. Physical activity and sports team participation: associations with academic outcomes in middle school and high school students. J Sch Health 2010;80(1):31–7.

19. Longmuir PE, Brothers JA, de Ferranti SD, et al. Promotion of physical activity for children and adults with congenital heart disease: a scientific statement from the American Heart Association. Circulation 2013;127(21):2147–59.

20. Rhodes J, Curran TJ, Camil L, et al. Sustained effects of cardiac rehabilitation in children with serious congenital heart disease. Pediatrics 2006;118(3): e586–93.

21. Rhodes J, Curran TJ, Camil L, et al. Impact of cardiac rehabilitation on the exercise function of children with serious congenital heart disease. Pediatrics 2005; 116(6):1339–45.

22. Fredriksen PM, Kahrs N, Blaasvaer S, et al. Effect of physical training in children and adolescents with congenital heart disease. Cardiol Young 2000; 10(2):107–14.

23. O'Byrne ML, Mercer-Rosa L, Ingall E, et al. Habitual exercise correlates with exercise performance in patients with conotruncal abnormalities. Pediatr Cardiol 2012;34(4):853–60.

24. Ubeda Tikkanen A, Opotowsky AR, Bhatt AB, et al. Physical activity is associated with improved aerobic exercise capacity over time in adults with congenital heart disease. Int J Cardiol 2013;168(5):4685–91.

25. Pahkala K, Heinonen OJ, Lagstrom H, et al. Vascular endothelial function and leisure-time physical activity in adolescents. Circulation 2008;118(23):2353–9.

26. Dean PN, Gillespie CW, Greene EA, et al. Sports participation and quality of life in adolescents and young adults with congenital heart disease. Congenit Heart Dis 2015;10(2):169–79.

27. Opic P, Utens EM, Cuypers JA, et al. Sports participation in adults with congenital heart disease. Int J Cardiol 2015;187:175–82.

28. van der Bom T, Winter MM, Knaake JL, et al. Long-term benefits of exercise training in patients with a systemic right ventricle. Int J Cardiol 2015;179: 105–11.

29. Johnson JN, Ackerman MJ. Competitive sports participation in athletes with congenital long QT syndrome. JAMA 2012;308(8):764–5.

30. Lampert R, Cannom D, Olshansky B. Safety of sports participation in patients with implantable cardioverter defibrillators: a survey of Heart Rhythm Society members. J Cardiovasc Electrophysiol 2006; 17(1):11–5.

31. Lampert R, Cannom D. Sports participation for athletes with implantable cardioverter-defibrillators should be an individualized risk–benefit decision. Heart Rhythm 2008;5(6):861–3.

32. Law IH, Shannon K. Implantable cardioverter-defibrillators and the young athlete: can the two coexist? Pediatr Cardiol 2012;33(3):387–93.

33. Asif IM, Price D, Fisher LA, et al. Stages of psychological impact after diagnosis with serious or potentially lethal cardiac disease in young competitive athletes: a new model. J Electrocardiol 2015;48(3):298–310.

34. Gow RM, Borghese MM, Honeywell CR, et al. Activity intensity during free-living activities in children and adolescents with inherited arrhythmia syndromes: assessment by combined accelerometer and heart rate monitor. Circ Arrhythm Electrophysiol 2013;6(5):939–45.

35. Koyak Z, Harris L, de Groot JR, et al. Sudden cardiac death in adult congenital heart disease. Circulation 2012;126(16):1944–54.

36. Pemberton VL, McCrindle BW, Barkin S, et al. Report of the National Heart, Lung, and Blood Institute's Working Group on obesity and other cardiovascular risk factors in congenital heart disease. Circulation 2010;121(9):1153–9.

37. Shustak RJ, McGuire SB, October TW, et al. Prevalence of obesity among patients with congenital and acquired heart disease. Pediatr Cardiol 2012;33(1):8–14.

38. Vaseghi M, Ackerman M, Mandapati R. Restricting sports for athletes with heart disease: are we saving lives, avoiding lawsuits, or just promoting obesity and sedentary living? Pediatr Cardiol 2012;33(3):407–16.

39. Mitchell JH, Maron BJ, Epstein SE. 16th Bethesda conference: cardiovascular abnormalities in the athlete: recommendations regarding eligibility for competition. October 3-5, 1984. J Am Coll Cardiol 1985;6(6):1186–232.

40. Wren C. Sudden death in children and adolescents. Heart 2002;88(4):426–31.

41. Diller GP, Kempny A, Alonso-Gonzalez R, et al. Survival prospects and circumstances of death in contemporary adult congenital heart disease patients under follow-up at a large tertiary centre. Circulation 2015;132(22):2118–25.

42. Silka MJ, Hardy BG, Menashe VD, et al. A population-based prospective evaluation of risk of sudden cardiac death after operation for common congenital heart defects. J Am Coll Cardiol 1998;32(1):245–51.

43. Gallego P, Gonzalez AE, Sanchez-Recalde A, et al. Incidence and predictors of sudden cardiac arrest in adults with congenital heart defects repaired before adult life. Am J Cardiol 2012;110(1):109–17.

44. Fletcher GF, Ades PA, Kligfield P, et al. Exercise standards for testing and training: a scientific statement from the American Heart Association. Circulation 2013;128(8):873–934.

45. La Gerche A, Gewillig M. What limits cardiac performance during exercise in normal subjects and in healthy Fontan patients? Int J Pediatr 2010. [Epub ahead of print].

46. Goldberg DJ, French B, McBride MG, et al. Impact of oral sildenafil on exercise performance in children and young adults after the Fontan operation: a randomized, double-blind, placebo-controlled, crossover trial. Circulation 2011;123(11):1185–93.

47. Douard H, Vuillemin C, Bordier P, et al. Normal blood-pressure profiles on effort according to age, sex and exercise protocols. Arch Mal Coeur Vaiss 1994;87(3):311–8 [in French].

48. Williams MA, Haskell WL, Ades PA, et al. Resistance exercise in individuals with and without cardiovascular disease: 2007 update - a scientific statement from the American Heart Association Council on Clinical Cardiology and Council on Nutrition, Physical Activity, and Metabolism. Circulation 2007;116(5):572–84.

49. Lawless CE. Sports cardiology essentials: evaluation, management, and case studies. New York: Springer; 2011.

50. Weiner RB, Baggish AL. Exercise-induced cardiac remodeling. Prog Cardiovasc Dis 2012;54(5):380–6.

51. Arbab-Zadeh A, Perhonen M, Howden E, et al. Cardiac remodeling in response to 1 year of intensive endurance training. Circulation 2014;130(24):2152–61.

52. Kovacs R, Baggish AL. Cardiovascular adaptation in athletes. Trends Cardiovasc Med 2016;26(1):46–52.

53. Duppen N, Takken T, Hopman MT, et al. Systematic review of the effects of physical exercise training programmes in children and young adults with congenital heart disease. Int J Cardiol 2013;168(3):1779–87.

54. Tikkanen AU, Oyaga AR, Riano OA, et al. Paediatric cardiac rehabilitation in congenital heart disease: a systematic review. Cardiol Young 2012;22(3):241–50.

55. Longmuir PE, Tremblay MS, Goode RC. Postoperative exercise training develops normal levels of physical activity in a group of children following cardiac surgery. Pediatr Cardiol 1990;11(3):126–30.

56. Singh TP, Curran TJ, Rhodes J. Cardiac rehabilitation improves heart rate recovery following peak exercise in children with repaired congenital heart disease. Pediatr Cardiol 2007;28(4):276–9.

57. Brown DW, Dipilato AE, Chong EC, et al. Sudden unexpected death after balloon valvuloplasty for congenital aortic stenosis. J Am Coll Cardiol 2010;56(23):1939–46.

58. Longmuir PE, McCrindle BW. Physical activity restrictions for children after the Fontan

operation: disagreement between parent, cardiologist, and medical record reports. Am Heart J 2009; 157(5):853–9.

59. Roston TM, De Souza AM, Sandor GG, et al. Physical activity recommendations for patients with electrophysiologic and structural congenital heart disease: a survey of Canadian health care providers. Pediatr Cardiol 2013;34(6):1374–81.

60. Paterick TE, Paterick TJ, Fletcher GF, et al. Medical and legal issues in the cardiovascular evaluation of competitive athletes. JAMA 2005;294(23):3011–8.

61. Panhuyzen-Goedkoop NM, Smeets JL. Legal responsibilities of physicians when making participation decisions in athletes with cardiac disorders: do guidelines provide a solid legal footing? Br J Sports Med 2014;48(15):1193–5.

62. Litwin PE, Eisenberg MS, Hallstrom AP, et al. The location of collapse and its effect on survival from cardiac arrest. Ann Emerg Med 1987;16(7):787–91.

63. de Vreede-Swagemakers JJ, Gorgels AP, Dubois-Arbouw WI, et al. Out-of-hospital cardiac arrest in the 1990's: a population-based study in the Maastricht area on incidence, characteristics and survival. J Am Coll Cardiol 1997;30(6):1500–5.

64. Valenzuela TD, Roe DJ, Nichol G, et al. Outcomes of rapid defibrillation by security officers after cardiac arrest in casinos. N Engl J Med 2000;343(17):1206–9.

65. Page RL, Joglar JA, Kowal RC, et al. Use of automated external defibrillators by a U.S. airline. N Engl J Med 2000;343(17):1210–6.

66. Marijon E, Bougouin W, Karam N, et al. Survival from sports-related sudden cardiac arrest: in sports facilities versus outside of sports facilities. Am Heart J 2015;170(2):339–45.e331.

67. Walsh EP. Sudden death in adult congenital heart disease: risk stratification in 2014. Heart Rhythm 2014;11(10):1735–42.

68. Moola F, Fusco C, Kirsh JA. The perceptions of caregivers toward physical activity and health in youth with congenital heart disease. Qual Health Res 2011;21(2):278–91.

69. Moola F, Faulkner GE, Kirsh JA, et al. Physical activity and sport participation in youth with congenital heart disease: perceptions of children and parents. Adapt Phys Activ Q 2008;25(1):49–70.

70. Levine BD, Baggish AL, Kovacs RJ, et al. Eligibility and disqualification recommendations for competitive athletes with cardiovascular abnormalities: task force 1: classification of sports: dynamic, static, and impact: a scientific statement from the American Heart Association and American College of Cardiology. J Am Coll Cardiol 2015;66(21):2350–5.

71. Diller GP, Giardini A, Dimopoulos K, et al. Predictors of morbidity and mortality in contemporary Fontan patients: results from a multicenter study including cardiopulmonary exercise testing in 321 patients. Eur Heart J 2010;31(24):3073–83.

72. Khairy P, Fernandes SM, Mayer JE Jr, et al. Long-term survival, modes of death, and predictors of mortality in patients with Fontan surgery. Circulation 2008;117(1):85–92.

73. Braverman AC, Harris KM, Kovacs RJ, et al. Eligibility and disqualification recommendations for competitive athletes with cardiovascular abnormalities: task force 7: aortic diseases, including Marfan syndrome: a scientific statement from the American Heart Association and American College of Cardiology. J Am Coll Cardiol 2015;66(21):2398–405.

74. Hatzaras I, Tranquilli M, Coady M, et al. Weight lifting and aortic dissection: more evidence for a connection. Cardiology 2007;107(2):103–6.

75. Malhotra R, Mistry D, Saunders C, et al. High prevalence of aortopathy and bicuspid aortic valve in elite intercollegiate athletes. J Am Coll Cardiol 2013; 61(10_S).

76. Fried TR. Shared decision making–finding the sweet spot. N Engl J Med 2016;374(2):104–6.

Exercise Prescription for the Athlete with Cardiomyopathy

Sara Saberi, MD, MS[a],*, Sharlene M. Day, MD[b]

KEYWORDS

- Cardiomyopathy • Sports participation • Exercise • Sudden cardiac death • Bethesda conference

KEY POINTS

- Current international guidelines recommend that athletes with cardiomyopathies refrain from all but low-intensity competitive sports independent of the presence or absence of high-risk features for sudden cardiac death (SCD).
- The incidence of SCD among athletes is low and not different than age-matched nonathlete populations. Among studies of SCD in athletes, the causes of death are widely discrepant. Hypertrophic cardiomyopathy is not uniformly the single most common cause of SCD in young athletes.
- Risk of SCD with sports participation is likely not equivalent for all athletes and many may be able to continue to compete safely. At present, risk stratification for SCD in athletes with cardiomyopathy is challenging and more data are needed before existing guidelines can be modified.

A question that care providers for patients with cardiomyopathies are often asked is "Can I exercise?" This question is not a simple one deserving of a "yes" or "no" answer. It becomes even more complicated when the patients posing the question are athletes, some of whom depend on their physical capabilities to make a living and almost all of whom depend on them to feel "alive" every day. So, how can one balance the patient's desire to exercise, train, and compete against a real or perceived risk of causing harm? Do these recommendations differ depending on the type of cardiomyopathy? What data inform existing guidelines? How should clinicians guide the new cohort of individuals who carry a gene mutation yet lack any evidence of clinical disease (genotype positive-phenotype negative)?

INHERITED CARDIOMYOPATHIES PRIMER
Hypertrophic Cardiomyopathy

Hypertrophic cardiomyopathy (HCM) is the most common genetic cardiovascular disease, affecting 1 in 500 people and characterized by ventricular hypertrophy and relaxation abnormalities.[1] It is inherited in an autosomal-dominant fashion and caused by mutations in cardiac sarcomere protein genes.[2] Despite being considered a monogenic disease, HCM is very heterogeneous with respect to clinical disease severity, even within a single family sharing an identical mutation. Diagnosis of HCM relies primarily on imaging informed by history and physical examination. Echocardiogram typically demonstrates a nondilated, hypertrophied, hyperdynamic left ventricle (LV) in the absence

Funding Sources: AHA Award 11CRP7510001, MICHR UL1TR000433 (S. Saberi); NIH R01 GRANT11572784 (S.M. Day).

Conflict of Interest: Nil.

[a] Division of Cardiovascular Medicine, Department of Internal Medicine, University of Michigan School of Medicine, Frankel Cardiovascular Center, Suite 2364, 1500 East Medical Center Drive, Ann Arbor, MI 48109-5853, USA; [b] Division of Cardiovascular Medicine, Department of Internal Medicine, University of Michigan School of Medicine, 1150 West Medical Center Drive, 7301 MSRBIII, Ann Arbor, MI 48109-5644, USA

* Corresponding author.

E-mail address: saberis@med.umich.edu

0733-8651/16/© 2016 Elsevier Inc. All rights reserved.

cardiology.theclinics.com

of any other disease that may otherwise explain the hypertrophy (**Fig. 1**). HCM can be complicated by sudden cardiac death (SCD), heart failure (HF), and/or cardioembolic stroke resulting from atrial fibrillation. Treatment options for HCM include implantable cardioverter-defibrillator (ICD) therapy to prevent SCD and medications, percutaneous alcohol septal ablation, or surgical myectomy to reduce symptomatic outflow tract obstruction. Many patients have a normal life expectancy, as the average mortality rate for individuals afflicted with HCM roughly equals that of the US population.[2]

Dilated Cardiomyopathy

Dilated cardiomyopathy (DCM) is characterized by dilation and impaired systolic function of the left or both ventricles (**Fig. 2**). DCM can present with symptomatic HF, arrhythmias, thromboembolic complications, or SCD. It may also be detected incidentally in asymptomatic individuals. Idiopathic DCM accounts for about 50% of patients with initially unexplained cardiomyopathy.[3] It is estimated that 20% to 35% of patients with idiopathic DCM have familial disease (FDC).[4–6] Most FDC is transmitted in an autosomal-dominant inheritance pattern. Several major societies and organizations have published guidelines for the treatment of HF with reduced ejection fraction that share many recommendations.[7–9]

Left Ventricle Noncompaction

LV noncompaction (LVNC) is newly recognized in its isolated form as a distinct cardiomyopathy. It is characterized by prominent LV trabeculae and deep intertrabecular recesses resulting in a double-layered myocardial structure consisting of an outer, compacted layer and inner, trabeculated or noncompacted layer (**Fig. 3**). Like HCM and DCM, autosomal-dominant inheritance is most common with reports of 12% to 50% having a family history of LVNC.[10–12] Its true incidence and prevalence are not known because of the lack of agreement on diagnostic criteria and the difficulty in its identification, and its heterogeneous clinical spectrum.

Its clinical expression is highly variable. Affected individuals may or may not have any symptoms, impaired systolic function and HF, arrhythmias, thromboembolic events, or sudden death.[11,13–16] The largest study on the natural history of children with LVNC highlights an overall mortality rate of nearly 13%, with systolic dysfunction and arrhythmias portending a worse prognosis.[14] Those with isolated hypertrabeculation and no associated systolic dysfunction, chamber dilation, or arrhythmias had a significantly decreased risk of mortality. A systematic review including five studies with a total of 241 adults with isolated LVNC also revealed an overall mortality rate of 14% over 39 months.[17]

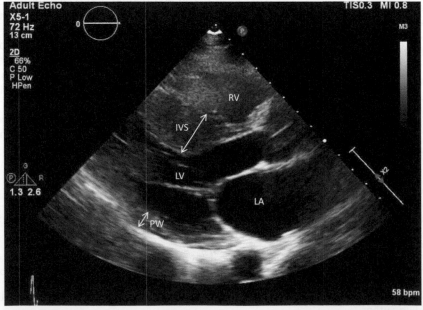

Fig. 1. Hypertrophic cardiomyopathy. Echocardiographic image of hypertrophic cardiomyopathy showing asymmetric hypertrophy of the interventricular septum (IVS) relative to the posterior wall (PW) (*double-headed arrows*). LA, left atrium; RV, right ventricle.

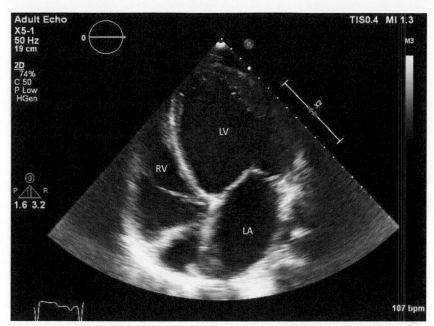

Fig. 2. Dilated cardiomyopathy. Echocardiographic image of dilated cardiomyopathy with dilated LV.

Arrhythmogenic Right Ventricular Cardiomyopathy

Arrhythmogenic right ventricular cardiomyopathy (ARVC) is characterized by fibrous or fatty replacement of the RV myocardium resulting in scarring and regional wall motion abnormalities and RV dilation (**Fig. 4**). It also involves the LV in a substantial number of cases. The desmosome is the primary source of genetic mutations.[18] Impaired desmosome function results in myocyte detachment and cell death when subjected to mechanical stress.

ARVC can present in a variety of ways, including palpitations, syncope, chest pain, dyspnea, and rarely, SCD. Clinical diagnosis is challenging and relies on a constellation of major and minor criteria many of which are based on advanced imaging modalities.[19] In a meta-analysis of 610 patients from 18 cohorts with ICDs, annualized rates of cardiac death, noncardiac death, and heart transplantation were 0.9%, 0.8%, and 0.9%, respectively.[20]

INCIDENCE OF SUDDEN CARDIAC DEATH IN ATHLETES

There is widespread agreement that SCD is the leading medical cause of death in athletes but its incidence is vigorously debated. Estimates of the incidence of SCD range from 1:917,000 athlete-years (AY) reported in Minnesota high school athletes[21] to 1:23,000 AY in a study of high schools with onsite automated external defibrillator (AED)

programs,[22] a difference of nearly 40-fold. Traditional estimates of SCD incidence in US athletes are usually approximately 1:200,000 AY,[23,24] although studies specifically examining college athletes show higher rates of SCD with a relatively consistent estimate of 1:43,000 to 1:67:000 AY.[25–28] The American Heart Association (AHA) recently reported an incidence of SCD in the United States of approximately 359,800 total cases annually in the general population.[29] The incidence of SCD among athletes is low and not different than age-matched nonathlete populations. In a national survey in France, the absolute number of SCDs associated with exertion in the general population (N = 770) far exceeds that observed among young competitive athletes (N = 50).[30] A Danish study reported a rate of SCD of 1:83,000 in athletes aged 12 to 35 versus a rate of SCD of 1:27,000 among nonathletes of the same age.[31] Most SCD events in athletes are caused by malignant arrhythmias, usually sustained ventricular tachycardia (VT) degenerating into ventricular fibrillation (VF), or primary VF itself, triggered by the physiologic demands of intense athletics. Such tragedies strike young athletes with cardiomyopathies, coronary artery anomalies, accessory pathways, or ion channel disorders.[32] Among those older than the age of 35 (masters athletes) advanced coronary atherosclerosis is the predominant cause of SCD during exercise.[33,34] Male athletes are consistently found to be at greater risk (by 9:1), and there seems to be a disproportionately higher risk among male

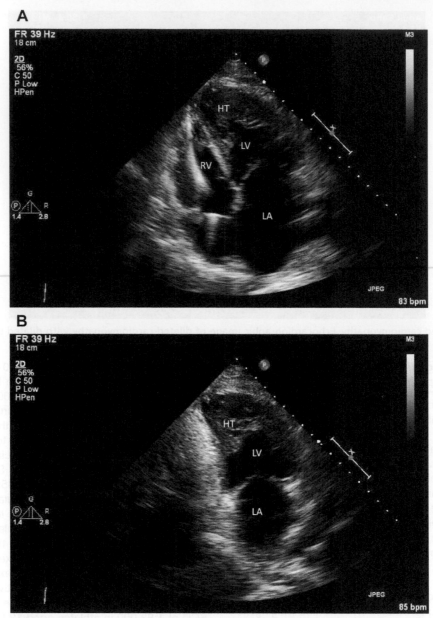

Fig. 3. Left ventricular noncompaction. (*A, B*) Echocardiographic images of LVNC showing hypertrabeculation (HT) in the LV apex.

African-American athletes.[35–37] Deaths in young competitive athletes are highly visible events fueled by media attention; however, more than 90% of all exercise-related SCDs occur in recreational athletes.[30,38]

RISK AND CAUSE OF SUDDEN CARDIAC DEATH IN ATHLETES WITH CARDIOMYOPATHY

Independent of sports participation, specific risk factors for SCD in patients with HCM include a prior history of VF, SCD, or sustained VT; family history of SCD in a first-degree family member younger than age 45; recent unexplained syncope; nonsustained VT; and massive hypertrophy greater than or equal to 30 mm.[39,40] Other potential risk factors include LV outflow tract obstruction, late gadolinium enhancement on cardiac MRI, LV apical aneurysm, certain genetic mutations, atrial fibrillation, and left atrial size.[41–45] An SCD risk prediction model has been developed incorporating many of these factors, allowing more individualized risk prediction.[46] HCM was

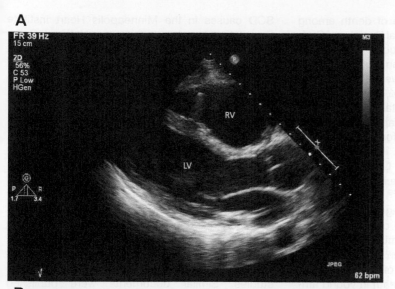

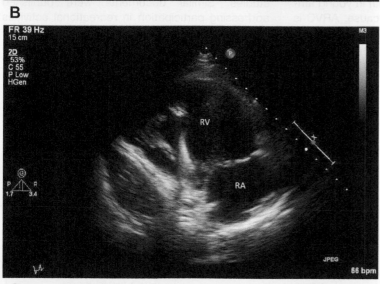

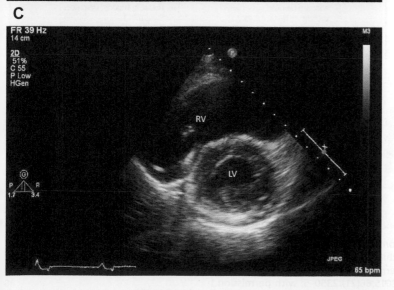

Fig. 4. Arrhythmogenic right ventricular cardiomyopathy. (*A–C*) Echocardiographic images of ARVC with RV dilation.

identified as the leading cause of death among young athletes by the US National Registry of Sudden Death in Athletes,[28,32,36] accounting for about one-third of the mortality in an autopsy-based athlete population.[32,35,36] However, HCM was found to be the cause of only 9% of SCD in young athletes in the Veneto region of Italy[47] and only 3% of SCD among National Collegiate Athletic Association athletes.[48] The reason for these discrepancies is not readily apparent.

Risk of SCD in FDC and LVNC has been shown to increase with the severity of LV systolic dysfunction and clinical HF.[14,49] Risk factors for SCD in ARVC include younger age, syncope, previous history of cardiac arrest or sustained VT, two or more disease-causing mutations, and LV involvement.[50–52] DCM has been identified as the cause of SCD in 3% to 17% of athletes.[32,36,48] Forensic registries of sudden death in young athletes do not include LVNC as a cause. ARVC is an important cause of SCD in young adults in the northern (Veneto) region of Italy, accounting for approximately 11% of cases overall and 22% in athletes[53,54] but only accounts for about 3% of

SCD causes in the Minneapolis Heart Institute Foundation registry and among National Collegiate Athletic Association athletes.[35,48] It is not clear whether this is caused by a higher overall prevalence of ARVC in this region of Italy, or underdiagnosis or misdiagnosis elsewhere.

GUIDELINES: BETHESDA AND BEYOND

The AHA, the American College of Cardiology (ACC; 36th Bethesda Conference), and the European Society of Cardiology (ESC) have developed consensus documents with recommendations for restriction from participation in competitive sports in trained athletes affected by a variety of genetic and acquired cardiovascular diseases.[55,56] These recommendations are in large part expert opinion given the lack of registry-based or randomized studies. Similar documents were published addressing participation in recreational activities and categorized safety of participation for the most common sports based on perceived levels of aerobic and anaerobic intensity (**Fig. 5**).[57,58] More recently, the AHA/ACC published an update

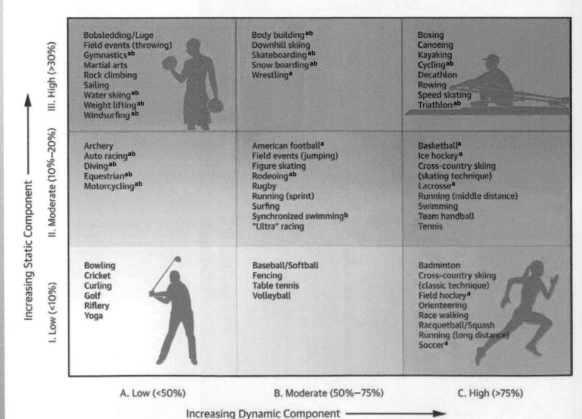

Fig. 5. Classification of sports. (*From* Levine BD, Baggish AL, Kovacs RJ, et al. Eligibility and disqualification recommendations for competitive athletes with cardiovascular abnormalities: task force 1: classification of sports: dynamic, static, and impact: a scientific statement from the American Heart Association and American College of Cardiology. J Am Coll Cardiol 2015;66(21):2350–5; with permission.)

to the prior Bethesda Conferences and recommendations are static in that a diagnosis of cardiomyopathy should preclude participation in competitive sports.[59] These recommendations are regardless of the individual's perceived risk of SCD based on disease severity or traditional risk factors. Despite these recommendations, many athletes have continued participation in competitive sports. In a survey of health behaviors among patients with HCM, 63% had participated in competitive athletics in their lifetime and 10% were still competing in at least one sport.[60] It is noteworthy that 60% believed that exercise restriction negatively affected their emotional well-being. One major difference between the European and American guidelines is that the ESC recommends exclusion for genotype positive–phenotype negative individuals from all competitive sports, with only leisure-time sporting activities recommended.[61] The Bethesda guidelines do not preclude these individuals from participation in competitive sports given a lack of evidence for adverse events.

Although the guidelines for competitive sports participation in cardiomyopathies have been largely static over the last 10 years, a drastic shift in the recommendations for sports participation for athletes with long-QT syndrome (LQTS) has occurred over the same time period. These guidelines now state that competitive sports participation may be considered after a comprehensive evaluation by a heart rhythm specialist, institution of treatment, and no symptoms for 3 months.[62] In a registry of 130 athletes with LQT1-3 genotypes with a mean follow-up of 5.1 years (663 AY), only one person experienced a sporting-related cardiac event (two appropriate VF-terminating ICD shocks).[63] In another series of 103 treatment-compliant children with LQTS participating in sports, there were no cardiac events or deaths related to sports participation in 755 patient-years of follow-up.[64] It should be noted that unlike LQTS where β-blockers have been shown to reduce arrhythmic event rates, it is unknown if β-blockers or other medications would have a similar benefit in cardiomyopathy patients. An ongoing multicenter registry of HCM and LQTS to evaluate the outcomes and quality of life over a range of physical activity levels, including vigorous exercise and competitive sports, will provide much needed data to inform future guideline documents for sports participation for the most common cardiomyopathy and arrhythmia syndrome, respectively.

Patients with cardiomyopathies deemed at high risk for SCD independent of sports participation will be recommended to have ICDs. Theoretically these should provide protection from SCD during sports, but concerns about device malfunction or injury have made experts reluctant to make different recommendations for sports participation for athletes with versus those without ICDs. However, new data have emerged that suggest that sports participation for athletes with ICDs may be safe. A prospective, multinational registry of 372 athletes with an ICD followed for a median of 31 months showed no deaths, resuscitated arrests, or defibrillation-related injuries during high-intensity competitive sports.[65] The most common heart disease represented among these athletes with an ICD was LQTS (73), followed by HCM (65), and ARVC (53). Thirty-one with DCM and five with LVNC also participated. A total of 21% of athletes received a shock from their device, 73% occurring during physical activity, 13% appropriate and 11% inappropriate. Only 1 out of 65 athletes with HCM received a shock during competition or practice, and 8 of 53 athletes with ARVC. Most athletes shocked during competition chose to continue playing subsequent to the shock. This study does raise the possibility that athletes may request an ICD be implanted so that they can continue to play sports. As providers, it is our duty to make responsible recommendations based on established guidelines for SCD risk stratification and not succumb to external pressures from athletes or sports organizations. Indeed, the guidelines state that ICDs should not be implanted for the sole purpose of permitting participation in high-intensity sports.[39,59]

The risk of SCD has dominated the discussion about sports participation for athletes with cardiomyopathies. However, there is also a theoretic risk of athletic training provoking or exacerbating the pathologic remodeling associated with these conditions. At the current time, circumstantial evidence for this possibility exists only for ARVC. Two studies of patients with ARVC (totaling 197 patients, 93 of whom were identified as endurance athletes by different definitions) suggest that endurance exercise increases disease penetrance, arrhythmic risk, and progression to HF.[66,67] The exercise ranges described in these studies are modest relative to competitive athletic training. Nonetheless, a dose-response relationship between composite exercise intensity and duration and disease progression and severity has been suggested.

APPROACH TO THE ATHLETE WITH CARDIOMYOPATHY

Although the updated guidelines still recommend exclusion of athletes with a cardiomyopathy from competitive sports, they do recognize patient autonomy with the following statement: "These recommendations do not strictly exclude in absolute terms fully informed athletes from participating in competitive athletic programs as long as such decision is ultimately made in concert with their physician and third-party interests."[59] This is an important step toward individualized decision making for athletes and their families. At this time, there is uncertainty as to whether continuing to play sports after a cardiomyopathy diagnosis increases an individual's risk of sudden death or whether withdrawal from sport participation lowers one's risk. Therefore, it seems appropriate to approach the athlete and members of his or her family and athletic team with a balanced discussion that incorporates available data, including gender, race, sport, and disease-specific factors that could influence risk. If they choose to continue to participate competitively, then the importance of team and staff preparedness and training in the case of an emergency should be emphasized, including the ready availability of AED at all practices and competitions. From a training perspective, the athlete and his or her coaches and trainers should design a program that builds good aerobic conditioning and ensures that the athlete stays well hydrated. The athlete should be advised of potential warning signs, such as dizziness, shortness of breath, or chest pain, which should be reported to their coaches immediately and cease practice or competition until further evaluation by the athletic trainers or physician.

Before beginning a training program, all patients with a confirmed cardiomyopathy diagnosis should have a comprehensive clinical evaluation, optimized pharmacologic therapy, and risk stratification. Before initiating the program a maximal, symptom, or peak volitional effort exercise test that simulates the level he or she will attain during their training and competition is an important component of the risk stratification. Expired gas exchange measurements are the most informative in that they allow an assessment of ventilatory abnormalities that are common in cardiomyopathies and are important for risk stratification.[68–71] Exercise-induced rhythm abnormalities and hypotension can be concerning findings that warrant further consideration before an exercise program can be safely recommended. Among athletes who have clear high-risk features where restriction from competition may be advisable, or among those who elect to abstain from competitive sports after their diagnosis, individualized exercise prescriptions for recreational exercise can be developed that incorporate parameters from the symptom-limited exercise test. Such exercise prescriptions should include information about frequency, intensity, duration, mode, and rate of progression. Exercise intensity should be equivalent to 50% to 80% of maximum capacity, using a combination of perceived exertion levels (targeting Borg scale levels between 12 and 14) and establishing target heart rate zones via the heart rate reserve method (Karvonen formula).

There is evidence that it may be safe for athletes with ICDs to exercise and compete.[65,72] Optimizing the pacemaker programming, including the upper rate limit and rate responsiveness, maximizes the patient's ability to perform. In patients with ICDs, it is prudent to keep the heart rate 20 beats per minute below the threshold of activation. There are a variety of wearable technologies available commercially that can help athletes monitor their heart rate during exercise and make real-time adjustments to their exercise intensity to maintain target heart rate zones. Heart monitors with chest straps are advisable because they are the most accurate. Given that most athletes with cardiomyopathies do not have an indication for ICD implantation, the AHA recommends that an AED be present at any school in which an emergency medical services call-to-shock time of 5 minutes or less cannot be achieved more than 90% of the time.[73] In addition to having the requisite equipment, every school or institution sponsoring athletic activities should have an emergency action plan that is developed in concert with local emergency medical services personnel and reviewed annually. Guidelines regarding specific conditioning recommendations and education and training requirements have been established.[74] Appropriate education and training should be made available to all involved personnel, including coaches, families, fellow athletes, and staff. Some athletes may even want to consider purchasing such a device on their own.

SUMMARY

The current understanding of cardiomyopathies and associated risk of SCD has evolved significantly over the past few decades and it is possible that such risk has been overestimated. Many athletes with cardiomyopathies choose to compete and enjoy all the physical and emotional benefits of athletics. Contemporary guidelines take a necessarily conservative approach to sports participation for athletes with cardiomyopathies because of a lack of evidence on which to base recommendations. International registries are now being established to help refine the guidelines with the hope that many athletes may be able to safely compete and enjoy the vast benefits of athletics.

REFERENCES

1. Maron BJ. Hypertrophic cardiomyopathy: a systematic review. JAMA 2002;287(10):1308–20.
2. Maron BJ, Maron MS. Hypertrophic cardiomyopathy. Lancet 2013;381(9862):242–55.
3. Felker GM, Thompson RE, Hare JM, et al. Underlying causes and long-term survival in patients with initially unexplained cardiomyopathy. N Engl J Med 2000;342(15):1077–84.
4. Goerss JB, Michels VV, Burnett J, et al. Frequency of familial dilated cardiomyopathy. Eur Heart J 1995; 16(Suppl O):2–4.
5. Grunig E, Tasman JA, Kucherer H, et al. Frequency and phenotypes of familial dilated cardiomyopathy. J Am Coll Cardiol 1998;31(1):186–94.
6. Michels VV, Moll PP, Miller FA, et al. The frequency of familial dilated cardiomyopathy in a series of patients with idiopathic dilated cardiomyopathy. N Engl J Med 1992;326(2):77–82.
7. Yancy CW, Jessup M, Bozkurt B, et al. ACCF/AHA guideline for the management of heart failure: executive summary: a report of the American College of Cardiology Foundation/American Heart Association Task Force on practice guidelines. Circulation 2013;128(16):1810–52.
8. McMurray JJ, Adamopoulos S, Anker SD, et al. ESC guidelines for the diagnosis and treatment of acute and chronic heart failure 2012: the task force for the diagnosis and treatment of acute and chronic heart failure 2012 of the European Society of Cardiology. Developed in collaboration with the Heart Failure Association (HFA) of the ESC. Eur Heart J 2012; 33(14):1787–847.
9. Lindenfeld J, Albert NM, Boehmer JP, et al. HFSA 2010 comprehensive heart failure practice guideline. J Card Fail 2010;16(6):e1–194.
10. Weiford BC, Subbarao VD, Mulhern KM. Noncompaction of the ventricular myocardium. Circulation 2004;109(24):2965–71.
11. Oechslin EN, Attenhofer Jost CH, Rojas JR, et al. Long-term follow-up of 34 adults with isolated left ventricular noncompaction: a distinct cardiomyopathy with poor prognosis. J Am Coll Cardiol 2000; 36(2):493–500.
12. Zaragoza MV, Arbustini E, Narula J. Noncompaction of the left ventricle: primary cardiomyopathy with an elusive genetic etiology. Curr Opin Pediatr 2007; 19(6):619–27.
13. Paterick TE, Tajik AJ. Left ventricular noncompaction: a diagnostically challenging cardiomyopathy. Circulation 2012;76(7):1556–62.
14. Brescia ST, Rossano JW, Pignatelli R, et al. Mortality and sudden death in pediatric left ventricular noncompaction in a tertiary referral center. Circulation 2013;127(22):2202–8.
15. Caliskan K, Michels M, Geleijnse ML, et al. Frequency of asymptomatic disease among family members with noncompaction cardiomyopathy. Am J Cardiol 2012;110(10):1512–7.
16. Greutmann M, Mah ML, Silversides CK, et al. Predictors of adverse outcome in adolescents and adults with isolated left ventricular noncompaction. Am J Cardiol 2012;109(2):276–81.
17. Bhatia NL, Tajik AJ, Wilansky S, et al. Isolated noncompaction of the left ventricular myocardium in adults: a systematic overview. J Card Fail 2011; 17(9):771–8.
18. Sen-Chowdhry S, Syrris P, McKenna WJ. Genetics of right ventricular cardiomyopathy. J Cardiovasc Electrophysiol 2005;16(8):927–35.
19. Marcus FI, McKenna WJ, Sherrill D, et al. Diagnosis of arrhythmogenic right ventricular cardiomyopathy/dysplasia: proposed modification of the task force criteria. Circulation 2010;121(13):1533–41.
20. Schinkel AF. Implantable cardioverter defibrillators in arrhythmogenic right ventricular dysplasia/cardiomyopathy: patient outcomes, incidence of appropriate and inappropriate interventions, and complications. Circ Arrhythm Electrophysiol 2013; 6(3):562–8.
21. Roberts WO, Stovitz SD. Incidence of sudden cardiac death in Minnesota High School athletes 1993-2012 screened with a standardized preparticipation evaluation. J Am Coll Cardiol 2013; 62(14):1298–301.
22. Drezner JA, Rao AL, Heistand J, et al. Effectiveness of emergency response planning for sudden cardiac arrest in United States high schools with automated external defibrillators. Circulation 2009; 120(6):518–25.
23. Maron BJ, Gohman TE, Aeppli D. Prevalence of sudden cardiac death during competitive sports activities in Minnesota high school athletes. J Am Coll Cardiol 1998;32(7):1881–4.
24. Maron BJ, Haas TS, Ahluwalia A, et al. Incidence of cardiovascular sudden deaths in Minnesota high school athletes. Heart Rhythm 2013;10(3):374–7.
25. Drezner JA, Rogers KJ, Zimmer RR, et al. Use of automated external defibrillators at NCAA Division I universities. Med Sci Sports Exerc 2005;37(9): 1487–92.
26. Harmon KG, Asif IM, Klossner D, et al. Incidence of sudden cardiac death in National Collegiate Athletic Association athletes. Circulation 2011;123(15): 1594–600.
27. Harmon KG, Asif IM, Maleszewski JJ, et al. Incidence, cause, and comparative frequency of sudden cardiac death in National Collegiate Athletic Association Athletes: a decade in review. Circulation 2015;132(1):10–9.

28. Maron BJ, Haas TS, Murphy CJ, et al. Incidence and causes of sudden death in U.S. college athletes. J Am Coll Cardiol 2014;63(16):1636–43.

29. Mozaffarian D, Benjamin EJ, Go AS, et al. Heart disease and stroke statistics-2016 update: a report from the American Heart Association. Circulation 2016;133(4):e38–60.

30. Marijon E, Tafflet M, Celermajer DS, et al. Sports-related sudden death in the general population. Circulation 2011;124(6):672–81.

31. Holst AG, Winkel BG, Theilade J, et al. Incidence and etiology of sports-related sudden cardiac death in Denmark: implications for preparticipation screening. Heart Rhythm 2010;7(10):1365–71.

32. Maron BJ, Doerer JJ, Haas TS, et al. Sudden deaths in young competitive athletes: analysis of 1866 deaths in the United States, 1980-2006. Circulation 2009;119(8):1085–92.

33. Virmani R, Robinowitz M, McAllister HA Jr. Nontraumatic death in joggers. A series of 30 patients at autopsy. Am J Med 1982;72(6):874–82.

34. Waller BF, Roberts WC. Sudden death while running in conditioned runners aged 40 years or over. Am J Cardiol 1980;45(6):1292–300.

35. Maron BJ. Sudden death in young athletes. N Engl J Med 2003;349(11):1064–75.

36. Maron BJ, Shirani J, Poliac LC, et al. Sudden death in young competitive athletes. Clinical, demographic, and pathological profiles. JAMA 1996;276(3):199–204.

37. Maron BJ, Carney KP, Lever HM, et al. Relationship of race to sudden cardiac death in competitive athletes with hypertrophic cardiomyopathy. J Am Coll Cardiol 2003;41(6):974–80.

38. Berdowski J, de Beus MF, Blom M, et al. Exercise-related out-of-hospital cardiac arrest in the general population: incidence and prognosis. Eur Heart J 2013;34(47):3616–23.

39. Gersh BJ, Maron BJ, Bonow RO, et al. ACCF/AHA guideline for the diagnosis and treatment of hypertrophic cardiomyopathy: a report of the American College of Cardiology Foundation/American Heart Association Task Force on Practice Guidelines. Circulation 2011;124(24):e783–831.

40. Maron BJ, McKenna WJ, Danielson GK, et al. American College of Cardiology/European Society of Cardiology clinical expert consensus document on hypertrophic cardiomyopathy. A report of the American College of Cardiology foundation task force on clinical expert consensus documents and the European Society of Cardiology Committee for Practice Guidelines. Eur Heart J 2003;24(21):1965–91.

41. Elliott PM, Gimeno JR, Tome MT, et al. Left ventricular outflow tract obstruction and sudden death risk in patients with hypertrophic cardiomyopathy. Eur Heart J 2006;27(16):1933–41.

42. Spirito P, Autore C, Rapezzi C, et al. Syncope and risk of sudden death in hypertrophic cardiomyopathy. Circulation 2009;119(13):1703–10.

43. Moon JC, McKenna WJ, McCrohon JA, et al. Toward clinical risk assessment in hypertrophic cardiomyopathy with gadolinium cardiovascular magnetic resonance. J Am Coll Cardiol 2003;41(9):1561–7.

44. Maron MS, Finley JJ, Bos JM, et al. Prevalence, clinical significance, and natural history of left ventricular apical aneurysms in hypertrophic cardiomyopathy. Circulation 2008;118(15):1541–9.

45. Watkins H, Rosenzweig A, Hwang DS, et al. Characteristics and prognostic implications of myosin missense mutations in familial hypertrophic cardiomyopathy. N Engl J Med 1992;326(17):1108–14.

46. O'Mahony C, Jichi F, Pavlou M, et al. A novel clinical risk prediction model for sudden cardiac death in hypertrophic cardiomyopathy (HCM Risk-SCD). Eur Heart J 2014;35(30):2010–20.

47. Corrado D, Basso C, Pavei A, et al. Trends in sudden cardiovascular death in young competitive athletes after implementation of a preparticipation screening program. JAMA 2006;296(13):1593–601.

48. Harmon KG, Drezner JA, Maleszewski JJ, et al. Pathogeneses of sudden cardiac death in national collegiate athletic association athletes. Circ Arrhythm Electrophysiol 2014;7(2):198–204.

49. Bardy GH, Lee KL, Mark DB, et al. Amiodarone or an implantable cardioverter-defibrillator for congestive heart failure. N Engl J Med 2005;352(3):225–37.

50. Corrado D, Leoni L, Link MS, et al. Implantable cardioverter-defibrillator therapy for prevention of sudden death in patients with arrhythmogenic right ventricular cardiomyopathy/dysplasia. Circulation 2003;108(25):3084–91.

51. Corrado D, Calkins H, Link MS, et al. Prophylactic implantable defibrillator in patients with arrhythmogenic right ventricular cardiomyopathy/dysplasia and no prior ventricular fibrillation or sustained ventricular tachycardia. Circulation 2010;122(12):1144–52.

52. Quarta G, Muir A, Pantazis A, et al. Familial evaluation in arrhythmogenic right ventricular cardiomyopathy: impact of genetics and revised task force criteria. Circulation 2011;123(23):2701–9.

53. Corrado D, Basso C, Schiavon M, et al. Screening for hypertrophic cardiomyopathy in young athletes. N Engl J Med 1998;339(6):364–9.

54. Corrado D, Fontaine G, Marcus FI, et al. Arrhythmogenic right ventricular dysplasia/cardiomyopathy: need for an international registry. Study Group on Arrhythmogenic Right Ventricular Dysplasia/Cardiomyopathy of the Working Groups on Myocardial and Pericardial Disease and Arrhythmias of the European Society of Cardiology and of the Scientific Council on Cardiomyopathies of the World Heart Federation. Circulation 2000;101(11):E101–6.

55. Maron BJ, Zipes DP. Introduction: eligibility recommendations for competitive athletes with cardiovascular abnormalities-general considerations. J Am Coll Cardiol 2005;45(8):1318–21.

56. Pelliccia A, Fagard R, Bjornstad HH, et al. Recommendations for competitive sports participation in athletes with cardiovascular disease: a consensus document from the Study Group of Sports Cardiology of the Working Group of Cardiac Rehabilitation and Exercise Physiology and the Working Group of Myocardial and Pericardial Diseases of the European Society of Cardiology. Eur Heart J 2005; 26(14):1422–45.

57. Maron BJ, Chaitman BR, Ackerman MJ, et al. Recommendations for physical activity and recreational sports participation for young patients with genetic cardiovascular diseases. Circulation 2004;109(22): 2807–16.

58. Pelliccia A, Corrado D, Bjornstad HH, et al. Recommendations for participation in competitive sport and leisure-time physical activity in individuals with cardiomyopathies, myocarditis and pericarditis. Eur J Cardiovasc Prev Rehabil 2006;13(6):876–85.

59. Maron BJ, Udelson JE, Bonow RO, et al. Eligibility and disqualification recommendations for competitive athletes with cardiovascular abnormalities: task force 3: hypertrophic cardiomyopathy, arrhythmogenic right ventricular cardiomyopathy and other cardiomyopathies, and myocarditis: a scientific statement from the American Heart Association and American College of Cardiology. Circulation 2015;132(22):e273–80.

60. Reineck E, Rolston B, Bragg-Gresham JL, et al. Physical activity and other health behaviors in adults with hypertrophic cardiomyopathy. Am J Cardiol 2013;111(7):1034–9.

61. Pelliccia A, Zipes DP, Maron BJ. Bethesda Conference #36 and the European Society of Cardiology consensus recommendations revisited a comparison of U.S. and European criteria for eligibility and disqualification of competitive athletes with cardiovascular abnormalities. J Am Coll Cardiol 2008; 52(24):1990–6.

62. Ackerman MJ, Zipes DP, Kovacs RJ, et al. Eligibility and disqualification recommendations for competitive athletes with cardiovascular abnormalities: task force 10: the cardiac channelopathies: a scientific statement from the American Heart Association and American College of Cardiology. Circulation 2015;132(22):e326–9.

63. Johnson JN, Ackerman MJ. Competitive sports participation in athletes with congenital long QT syndrome. JAMA 2012;308(8):764–5.

64. Aziz PF, Sweeten T, Vogel RL, et al. Sports participation in genotype positive children with long QT syndrome. JACC Clin Electrophysiol 2015;1(1–2): 62–70.

65. Lampert R, Olshansky B, Heidbuchel H, et al. Safety of sports for athletes with implantable cardioverter-defibrillators: results of a prospective, multinational registry. Circulation 2013;127(20):2021–30.

66. James CA, Bhonsale A, Tichnell C, et al. Exercise increases age-related penetrance and arrhythmic risk in arrhythmogenic right ventricular dysplasia/cardiomyopathy-associated desmosomal mutation carriers. J Am Coll Cardiol 2013;62(14):1290–7.

67. Saberniak J, Hasselberg NE, Borgquist R, et al. Vigorous physical activity impairs myocardial function in patients with arrhythmogenic right ventricular cardiomyopathy and in mutation positive family members. Eur J Heart Fail 2014;16(12):1337–44.

68. Myers J, Froelicher VF. Hemodynamic determinants of exercise capacity in chronic heart failure. Ann Intern Med 1991;115(5):377–86.

69. Myers J, Salleh A, Buchanan N, et al. Ventilatory mechanisms of exercise intolerance in chronic heart failure. Am Heart J 1992;124(3):710–9.

70. Finocchiaro G, Haddad F, Knowles JW, et al. Cardiopulmonary responses and prognosis in hypertrophic cardiomyopathy: a potential role for comprehensive noninvasive hemodynamic assessment. JACC Heart Fail 2015;3(5):408–18.

71. Coats CJ, Rantell K, Bartnik A, et al. Cardiopulmonary exercise testing and prognosis in hypertrophic cardiomyopathy. Circ Heart Fail 2015;8(6):1022–31.

72. Belardinelli R, Capestro F, Misiani A, et al. Moderate exercise training improves functional capacity, quality of life, and endothelium-dependent vasodilation in chronic heart failure patients with implantable cardioverter defibrillators and cardiac resynchronization therapy. Eur J Cardiovasc Prev Rehabil 2006;13(5):818–25.

73. Guidelines 2000 for cardiopulmonary resuscitation and emergency cardiovascular care. Part 4: the automated external defibrillator: key link in the chain of survival. The American Heart Association in Collaboration with the International Liaison Committee on Resuscitation. Circulation 2000;102(8 Suppl):I60–76.

74. Casa DJ, Anderson SA, Baker L, et al. The inter-association task force for preventing sudden death in collegiate conditioning sessions: best practices recommendations. J Athl Train 2012;47(4):477–80.

Beyond the Bruce Protocol
Advanced Exercise Testing for the Sports Cardiologist

Satyam Sarma, MD[a,b], Benjamin D. Levine, MD[a,b],*

KEYWORDS

- Exercise • Bruce protocol • Sports cardiology • V_{O_2}

KEY POINTS

- The Bruce protocol is not an optimal test for many athletes; rather, exercise testing should aim to recreate the exact circumstances during which symptoms arise.
- Lactate measurement during exercise can provide valuable information regarding the athlete's trained status for his or her event and help to exclude deconditioning from the differential.
- Understanding the physiology involved in specific sports is important in assessing an athlete's performance.

 Video content accompanies this article at http://www.cardiology.theclinics.com.

INTRODUCTION

For many clinicians, the Bruce protocol has become synonymous with exercise testing. Since its inception in 1950 to its evolution into the familiar 3-minute incremental stages by 1963, the protocol has quickly become the most common clinical treadmill exercise test.[1,2] A number of prognostic algorithms based on performance during the Bruce have been developed to inform clinicians on cardiac risk and prognosis, as well as functional capacity.[3–5] In this regard, the Bruce protocol has become the "go to" choice for the evaluation of exertional dyspnea.

When working with athletes, however, the Bruce protocol is rarely an optimal test because the goals for athletic testing are often different from the general public. In athletes, the purpose of testing is typically done to:

i. Evaluate baseline fitness and prescribe an exercise program or training zones;
ii. Evaluate continued progress after engaging in exercise training over a period of time;
iii. Diagnose cardiopulmonary conditions affecting exercise performance; and
iv. Provoke arrhythmias or evaluate hemodynamic response to exercise in an athlete with a known cardiovascular condition to determine whether it is safe to participate in competitive sports.

The key is to design a protocol that can safely and accurately answer these questions but is also tailored to the athlete's sport. Relying on a

The authors have nothing to disclose.
a Institute for Exercise and Environmental Medicine, Texas Health Presbyterian Hospital, 7232 Greenville Avenue, Dallas, TX 75231, USA; b Department of Internal Medicine, University of Texas Southwestern Medical Center, 5232 Harry Hines Boulevard, Dallas, TX 75390, USA
* Corresponding author. Institute for Exercise and Environmental Medicine, Texas Health Presbyterian Hospital, 7232 Greenville Avenue, Dallas, TX 75231.
E-mail address: BenjaminLevine@Texashealth.org

Cardiol Clin 34 (2016) 603–608
http://dx.doi.org/10.1016/j.ccl.2016.06.009
0733-8651/16/© 2016 Elsevier Inc. All rights reserved.

"one size fits all" approach can result in an inappropriate test that gives false reassurance to both the athlete and clinician. This review recommends strategies in designing appropriate and relevant tests to answer athlete questions and provides examples of exercise testing in a variety of sporting disciplines.

GRADED EXERCISE TESTING

The graded exercise test should be familiar to most sports clinicians and consists of incremental increases in workload by varying speed, elevation or both. The standard Bruce protocol starts at 1.7 miles per hour at 10° inclination and increases elevation by 2° and speed by approximately 1 mph every 3 minutes. From completion of the first stage at 4 metabolic equivalents, each successive stage increases workload by approximately 3 metabolic equivalents. The quantum jumps in aerobic workload between stages are relatively large for patients with heart disease which makes it a suboptimal test even for patients let alone for athletes. Moreover, it relies much more on steep grades for driving up the work requirements, which for many athletes are uncomfortable and for competitive athletes often cannot elicit a true maximal effort.

A number of other graded exercise tests take a different approach from the Bruce. Rather than varying both speed and elevation, protocols such as the Naughton (2 mph) or Balke (3 mph) keep speed constant and shorten stage duration with elevation increasing by either 3.5% or 2.5% during each 2-minute stage. Although low speed, these protocols provide 1-metabloc equivalent quanta between stages, which make them especially valuable for patients. For an athlete trying to accurately determine heart rate training zones and continued progress from training, using an exercise protocol with higher resolution helps to define aerobic training parameters, although of course faster speeds will be required than are available in "standard" clinical protocols. In particular, when identifying ventilatory thresholds, the Bruce protocol will often underestimate this important aerobic measurement compared with graded exercise tests that have smaller increases in workload between stages.[6]

To account for the increased aerobic capacity of an athlete, a number of protocols have modified the treadmill speed. Protocols such as the Astrand (5 mph) or Astrand-Saltin (variable)[7] pick a relatively high speed and increase elevation by 2° in 2-minute stages. This still allows for 1-metabolic equivalent differences between stages and, because of high speed, shortens the test to 10 to 12 minutes. Picking the fixed treadmill speed is subjective but can usually be accurately estimated by having the athlete run at a pace that can be easily sustained for 30 minutes. It does not matter if this speed is 6 mph (10 min/mile pace) or 10 mph (6 min/mile/pace); picking a comfortable running speed and then only changing grade is essential for testing athletes.

At the end of the graded exercise test to exhaustion, the athlete should know his or her maximal aerobic power (can be estimated by treadmill protocol—ie, calculated from horizontal and vertical work—if breath-by-breath gas exchange is not available), maximal heart rate and as well as ventilatory threshold if breath-by-breath gas exchange system is available or by the Conconi method (ie, heart rate break point) if no gas exchange system is present.[8] Graded exercise testing can also be useful for detecting exercise or catecholaminergic arrhythmias and ischemia.

NONGRADED EXERCISE TESTING

Athletes rarely perform graded aerobic exercise to exhaustion. Rather, many events require sustaining relatively fixed workloads over short or long durations of sport, whereas other events require sudden bursts of high-intensity exercise followed by lull periods. Recreating the circumstances involved in performance limitations in a sporting event can be difficult and requires creative thinking. If an athlete develops fatigue in the last kilometer of a 5K race, the test needs to recreate the whole race. Similarly if a football player (American style) has shortness of breath between plays, the test needs to incorporate high-intensity intervals separated periods of rest.

Although recreating conditions for a cross-country running or paced endurance event is relatively straightforward, reproducing sports that have periodic bursts of aerobic power are more challenging. In designing a testing protocol, the first step is to discuss with the athlete what symptoms are to be reproduced and when during the event they occur (**Fig. 1**). **Table 1** gives suggested frameworks for individual sports types, which can be used as a basis for designing the exercise protocol. Sports such as American style football or ice hockey require high degrees of exertion above lactate threshold, when lactate production exceeds clearance mechanisms and the skeletal muscles rely primarily on substrate-level phosphorylation. In these sports, a dedicated test of anaerobic capacity, such as a Wingate protocol,[9] or accumulated oxygen deficit (Medbo[10]) can be helpful in identifying limitations in substrate level capacity, although such tests are generally more

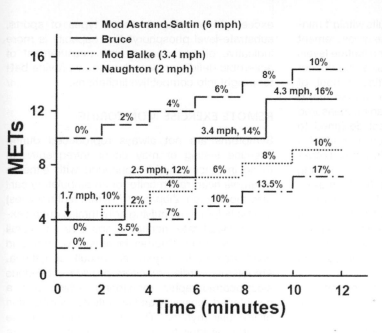

Fig. 1. Examples of various exercise testing protocols. The Naughton, modified Balke, and modified Astrand-Saltin keep speed constant and change incline every 2 minutes. The Bruce protocol changes both speed and incline every 3 minutes. The starting speed of the modified Astrand-Saltin protocol can be individualized to start at a speed below lactate threshold. In the example, a starting speed of 6 mph roughly corresponds to 10 METs and increases every 2 minutes by 1 MET, reaching 15 METs at 10% inclination. MET, metabolic equivalent.

useful for characterizing performance than they are for diagnosing sport specific exercise tolerance. Similarly, exercise economy is an additional tool to evaluate performance (measured by quantifying the relationship between steady-state speeds and Vo_2) in middle distance events and along with the measurement of Vo_{2max} allows the calculation of velocity at Vo_{2max}, which is closely associated with 5K speed.[11] Ultimately, it is important to understand the aerobic and anaerobic demands unique to an individual sport. The objective here, again, is to best reproduce the scenario and aerobic loads in which the athlete develops symptoms and can be modified as necessary depending on available exercise testing equipment (Videos 1 and 2).

Ideally, exercise testing modalities should also mimic the actual movements of the athlete's sport.

For sports such as ice hockey, inline roller blades can be used on a treadmill with a safety harness and overhead pulley system to prevent falls. For sports like basketball or football that require jumping, box jumping can be intermixed with treadmill testing. If testing facilities are not equipped or able to accommodate such exercises, a standard cycle ergometer can be used to reproduce the aerobic and heart rate profile of a sport with rapid changes in work rate. An important caveat with cycle testing is that not all athletes will be cycle trained and thus may underestimate performance.

Blood lactate levels are an important measurement during nongraded tests, which can provide insight into the conditioning state of the athlete relative to the demands of the sport. There are a number of commercially available handheld lactate monitors that can sample a pinprick or

Table 1
Suggested nongraded exercise testing protocols for various sports

Sport	Exercise Protocol
Ice hockey	High intensity (>90%–95% heart rate max) intervals for 90 s with 90 s rest between bouts repeated 6–10 times
American style football	Very high intensity (>95% heart rate max) intervals for 10 s with 30 s rest between bouts repeated 10–15 times
Football/soccer	Sustained moderate intensity effort (50%–70% heart rate max) for 2–3 min with 30–60 s of high-intensity effort (>90% heart rate max) repeated 10–15 times
Basketball	Box jumps 3–5 times as quickly as possible followed by moderate level intensity (60%–70% heart rate max) intervals for 1 min repeated 10–15 times
Triathlon	Swimming (if available) 45 min, cycling for 45 min, and running for 45 min

finger stick of blood and return results within 1 minute. This allows for rapid, real-time measurement while the athlete is exercising. Blood lactate levels should be measured at rest as well as no sooner than 2 to 3 minutes after starting a bout of steady-state exercise to allow for muscle metabolic kinetics to stabilize. Levels can be measured either with a steady-state protocol designed to mimic competition or can be used as part of a ramp protocol to define an athlete's lactate breakpoint. The increase in blood lactate from a resting baseline is termed the *lactate threshold*. As exercise intensity increases, lactate levels increase more rapidly and is termed the *lactate breakpoint* or *onset of blood lactate*. The exact breakpoint can be difficult to identify and many exercise physiology laboratories will use a cut point of 4 mmol/L.[12]

Compared with Vo_{2max}, athletic performance in longer duration endurance events such as the marathon is often better correlated with the Vo_2 at the lactate threshold,[13] although such correlations with performance depends on the duration of the sporting event. For example, a [La] threshold will be most relevant for efforts that last in the 2 to 3 hour range. In contrast, efforts that last 8 to 20 minutes will be more closely linked to Vo_2 max, and efforts that last less than 1 to 2 minutes depend more on power output and [La] tolerance than the Vo_2 and [La] threshold.[14]

For steady-state endurance events greater than 20 to 30 minutes, lactate levels in a well-trained individual should remain below the onset of blood lactate level (3–4 mmol/L) during exercise reflecting balance between lactate generation and efficient clearance within the body. In highly trained individuals, the lactate threshold can be close to 90% of Vo_{2max}. If lactate levels are above threshold during a simulated sports event, this may suggest that the athlete may be overestimating his or her capabilities, as may occur when transitioning from a lower to a higher level of competition (eg, high school to collegiate). Increasing a running pace from 5 min/miles to less than 5 may be the difference between running just below lactate threshold to crossing it. Alternatively, an elevated lactate threshold could also just signify that an athlete needs more sport and distance specific training to improve performance.

Blood lactate can also be measured during a graded test to define a break point.

For sports with bursts of high aerobic intensity, interpretation of blood lactate levels can be difficult. After a short bout of peak exertion, blood lactate levels will not peak for at least 2 to 3 minutes after exercise and in some types of athletes (eg, sprint or middle distance runners may reach or exceed 20 mmol/L). In these types of sports, substrate-level phosphorylation capacity is more indicative of performance and measurement of anaerobic deficit, as described, may provide better insight into competitive limitations.

REMOTE EXERCISE MONITORING

Symptoms are not always reproduced during exercise testing or may occur infrequently. In these instances, heart monitoring with either a wearable heart rate monitor or an ambulatory cardiac monitor (eg, Ziopatch, iRhythm technologies) can be helpful in identifying arrhythmias during exercise. Heart rate monitor straps give an overall heart rate trend. Sudden increases or jumps in heart rate could signify an occult arrhythmia. Ambulatory cardiac monitors provide continuous electrocardiographic monitoring, which has a heightened sensitivity and specificity for detection of irregular rhythms. The disadvantage to these monitors is their finite recording time, anywhere between 48 hours up to 4 weeks. An alternative approach is a commercially available solution, Alivecor, which provides an electrocardiograph on a smartphone using a modified smartphone case. Once purchased, the device can be used an infinite number of times. The recording quality is good but only if taken while at rest or motionless. The athlete should be instructed to have the device close by during training (either with a coach or trainer) and at the onset of symptoms, quickly record a tracing, save it, and send to his or her physician.

CASE STUDY

Here we describe a case of an Ironman triathlete who reported significant shortness of breath during his most recent races to illustrate the approaches to exercise testing in such a complex event. The subject was 49 years old and had competed in 9 triathlons (5 Ironmans). He noticed he had developed shortness of breath and persistent cough during the cycling portion of the event in 2 out of the last 4 races and was concerned about possible pulmonary edema limiting his performance. He ingested a large salt load before his most recent races and was worried this was causing pulmonary congestion.

We designed a protocol that involved 60 minutes of swimming (2.5 mph) and 90 minutes of cycling at 185 W. Blood lactates were measured every 30 minutes along with continuous heart rhythm monitoring. Serum cardiac biomarkers (brain natriuretic peptide and high-sensitivity cardiac troponin) were also measured at rest and immediately after the test. We used B-mode ultrasound imaging to assess for the presence of pulmonary congestion noninvasively by measuring "comet tails," essentially linear bundles of hyperechogenic signal emanating from the pleural reflection.[15]

After completion of the protocol, the patient denied any symptoms. He reported no cough or shortness of breath. Blood lactate after swimming was 2.0 mmol/L and after cycling was 3.6 mmol/L. Serum cardiac biomarkers were slightly elevated with high-sensitivity troponin of 0.037 ng/mL after exercise (upper limit of normal, 0.036 ng/mL) with serum brain natriuretic peptide essentially unchanged (12–15 ng/mL). There was evidence of mild subclinical pulmonary edema with a total of 7 "comet tails" in one-quarter of the lung zones queried. The significant of these comet tails is unclear in an asymptomatic person. Prior reports suggest up to 75% of triathletes develop some degree of pulmonary edema during races.[16]

Although a definitive etiology for the triathlete's intermittent episodes of coughing paroxysms and shortness of breath was not found, the testing protocol reassured him that there were no gross abnormalities in cardiac or respiratory function. This example illustrates the challenges in designing exercise protocols that best recapitulate cardiovascular and aerobic load of specific sporting events.

A second case occurred with an elite rower who and an electrocardiograph that was possibly suggestive of the long QT syndrome and had a syncopal episode after standing up to carry the boat back to the boat house after a competition. There was no structural heart disease and no family history of syncope or sudden cardiac death. The athlete was being held out of a critical national competition until the case could be resolved. We performed a simulated 2000-meter rowing race on a rowing ergometer with an "all-out" high-intensity start, followed by a base stroke rate chosen by the athlete for approximately 1000 meters with a final high-intensity 500-meter finish. We then had the athlete stand up and simulate a boat carry across the laboratory. This simulation reproduced an arrhythmia and syncope—however, rather than torsade de pointe, the patient had a narrow complex supraventricular tachycardia with postexercise hypotension. This arrhythmia was easily ablated, genetic testing revealed no known channelopathy and the athlete was cleared to play, ultimately winning an Olympic medal. This case illustrates how important it is to reproduce the exact demands of a sport and condition under which symptoms occurred.

SUMMARY

Graded exercise tests are the most common clinically used exercise protocols for testing athletes. However a "usual" clinical Bruce protocol is inappropriate and will likely be unrevealing for the majority of competitive athletes. The ability to perform sport specific protocols is absolutely essential for evaluating athletes and will be a more informative test for both the athlete and sports cardiologist. Considerable thought needs to be given in the design of a sports specific protocol, namely, (1) when during the event do symptoms occur (2) is the necessary testing equipment available to recreate the sport and (3) if not, can the aerobic power profile of the sport be recreated on what testing equipment is available? An understanding of the unique nature of the athlete's event is essential to the design, interpretation, and counseling of an advanced exercise test.

SUPPLEMENTARY DATA

Supplementary data related to this article can be found at http://dx.doi.org/10.1016/j.ccl.2016.06.009.

REFERENCES

1. Bruce RA, Blackmon JR, Jones JW, et al. Exercising testing in adult normal subjects and cardiac patients. Pediatrics 1963;32(Suppl):742–56.
2. Stuart RJ Jr, Ellestad MH. National survey of exercise stress testing facilities. Chest 1980;77:94–7.
3. Shaw LJ, Peterson ED, Shaw LK, et al. Use of a prognostic treadmill score in identifying diagnostic coronary disease subgroups. Circulation 1998;98: 1622–30.
4. Mark DB, Hlatky MA, Harrell FE Jr, et al. Exercise treadmill score for predicting prognosis in coronary artery disease. Ann Intern Med 1987;106: 793–800.
5. Heyward VH. Advance fitness assessment & exercise prescription. 3rd edition. Dallas (TX): The Cooper Institute for Aerobics Research; 1998.
6. Kang J, Chaloupka EC, Mastrangelo MA, et al. Physiological comparisons among three maximal treadmill exercise protocols in trained and untrained individuals. Eur J Appl Physiol 2001;84:291–5.
7. Astrand PO, Saltin B. Oxygen uptake during the first minutes of heavy muscular exercise. J Appl Physiol 1961;16:971–6.
8. Conconi F, Grazzi G, Casoni I, et al. The Conconi test: methodology after 12 years of application. Int J Sports Med 1996;17:509–19.
9. Bar-Or O. The Wingate anaerobic test. an update on methodology, reliability and validity. Sports Med 1987;4:381–94.

10. Medbo JI, Mohn AC, Tabata I, et al. Anaerobic capacity determined by maximal accumulated O2 deficit. J Appl Physiol 1988;64:50–60.

11. Levine BD, Stray-Gundersen J. "Living high-training low": effect of moderate-altitude acclimatization with low-altitude training on performance. J Appl Physiol (1985) 1997;83:102–12.

12. Sjodin B, Jacobs I. Onset of blood lactate accumulation and marathon running performance. Int J Sports Med 1981;2:23–6.

13. Coyle EF, Coggan AR, Hopper MK, et al. Determinants of endurance in well-trained cyclists. J Appl Physiol (1985) 1988;64:2622–30.

14. Levine BD. VO2max: what do we know, and what do we still need to know? J Physiol 2008;586:25–34.

15. Agricola E, Bove T, Oppizzi M, et al. "Ultrasound comet-tail images": a marker of pulmonary edema: a comparative study with wedge pressure and extravascular lung water. Chest 2005;127: 1690–5.

16. Pingitore A, Garbella E, Piaggi P, et al. Early subclinical increase in pulmonary water content in athletes performing sustained heavy exercise at sea level: ultrasound lung comet-tail evidence. Am J Physiol Heart Circ Physiol 2011;301: H2161–7.

Special Articles

Quick Evidence Synopsis
Coronary Artery Revascularization in Patients with Acute Coronary Syndrome and Comorbid Renal Disease

Date: June 15, 2015
Authors: Steven Lascher, DVM, PhD, MPH and David R. Goldmann, MD

What is the clinical question?

What are the benefits and harms of coronary artery revascularization in patients with acute coronary syndrome (ACS) and comorbid renal disease?

What does the evidence conclude?
What are the parameters of our evidence search?
What is the basis for the conclusion(s)?

Intervention	Quality of Evidence	Balance Between Benefits and Harms
Early revascularization vs medical treatment	Low	Tradeoff between benefits and harms

Quality of evidence: Quality of evidence scale (GRADE): high, moderate, low, and very low. For more information on the GRADE rating system, see http://www.gradeworkinggroup.org/index.htm.

Balance between benefits and harms: The Guideline Elements Model: beneficial, likely to be beneficial, unknown effectiveness, trade-off between benefits and harms, likely harmful, and harmful. For more information, see http://gem.med.yale.edu/default.htm.

Population: Adults with ACS and comorbid renal disease; renal disease severity

Population	Adults with ACS and comorbid renal disease Patient characteristics: demographics, family history of coronary artery disease (CAD), baseline cardiovascular risk profile (eg, Framingham risk profile), alcohol use, physical activity, diabetes, body mass index, other comorbidities, frailty Severity and duration of symptoms, prior angina, angiography stenosis location and degree Renal disease severity and duration Concomitant treatments
Intervention	Percutaneous coronary intervention (PCI; stent type and number) Coronary artery bypass graft (CABG) Location of revascularization: left main CAD, non-left main Combined procedures
Comparator	Active comparators
Primary outcome(s)	Mortality (all cause) All harms, including bleeding and infection

Settings: Inpatient
Intervention: Coronary artery revascularization by PCI or CABG
Comparator: Medical management
Outcome: Mortality (**Table 1**)

Cardiol Clin 34 (2016) 609–613
http://dx.doi.org/10.1016/j.ccl.2016.08.001
0733-8651/16

Table 1
Medical management versus revascularization in patients with coronary artery syndrome by GFRs

Outcome (Mortality, All-cause, by GFR)	Assumed Risk[a] Medical Therapy (95% CI)	Corresponding Risk[a] Early Revascularization (95% CI)	Odds Ratio[b] NNT (95% CI)	Number of Participants (Studies)	Confidence in the Effect Estimates (GRADE)	Comments
0–90 mL/min/1.73 m²						
Short-term mortality[c]	140/1000 (120–160)	107/1000 (90–130)	0.68 (0.54–0.84) 13 (7–104)	8229 (6 prospective observational and retrospective studies)[1]	Low	Favors early revascularization
One-year mortality	61/1000 (47–78)	550/1000 (519–581)	0.43 (0.20–0.94)	19,800 (4 prospective observational and retrospective studies)[1]	Low	Favors early revascularization
0–60 mL/min/1.73 m²						
Short-term mortality	273/1000 (251–295)	107/1000 (92–123)	0.69 (0.56–0.87) 4 (3–5)	6077 (5 prospective observational and retrospective studies)[1]	Low	Favors early revascularization
One-year mortality	304/1000 (290–320)	137/1000 (120–150)	0.4 (0.35–0.45) 4 (3–5)	8980 (3 prospective observational and retrospective studies)[1]	Low	Favors early revascularization
Two-year mortality	387/1000 (366–408)	271/1000 (243–298)	0.55 (0.34–0.90) 7 (6–12)	3066 (2 prospective observational and retrospective studies)[1]	Low	Favors early revascularization

	Control risk[a]	Intervention risk[a]	Relative effect (95% CI)[b] NNT	No. of participants (studies)	Quality (GRADE)	Comments
Three-year mortality	458/1000 (436–480)	328/1000 (299–356)	0.54 (0.31–0.96) 5 (4–7)	3066 (2 prospective observational and retrospective studies)[1]	Low	Favors early revascularization
0–30 mL/min/1.73 m²						
Short-term mortality	148/1000 (127–172)	91/1000 (74–111)	0.69 (0.53–0.90) 7 (5–15)	3673 (3 prospective observational and retrospective studies)[1]	Low	Favors early revascularization
One-year mortality	441/1000 (416–465)	237/1000 (199–276)	0.56 (0.44–0.72) 4 (3.7–5.5)	2059 (3 prospective observational and retrospective studies)[1]	Low	Favors early revascularization
0–15 mL/min/1.73 m²/dialysis						
One-year mortality	454/1000 (425–483)	241/1000 (199–282)	0.6 (0.46–0.80) 4 (3.6–5)	1546 (3 prospective observational and retrospective studies)[1]	Low	Favors early revascularization

Abbreviations: CI, confidence interval; GFR, glomerular filtration rate; GRADE, Grading of Recommendations Assessment, Development and Evaluation; NNT, number needed to treat.

[a] Illustrative comparative risks.
[b] All are calculated using random effects model.
[c] Short-term mortality is defined as in-hospital or 30-day mortality.[1]

What do clinical guidelines say?

Guideline for Percutaneous Coronary Intervention. A Report of the American College of Cardiology Foundation/American Heart Association Task Force on Practice Guidelines and the Society for Cardiovascular Angiography and Interventions, 2011.[2] (AGREE II Score: 81%)

This guideline does not provide specific recommendations about revascularization in patients with chronic kidney disease (CKD), but includes the following recommendations about avoiding contrast nephropathy in patients undergoing coronary angiographic procedures:

- In patients with CKD (creatinine clearance <60 mL/min), the volume of contrast media should be minimized. (Recommendation: I; Level of evidence: B)
- In patients undergoing PCI, the glomerular filtration rate (GFR) should be estimated, and the dosage of medications that are cleared by the kidney should be adjusted. (Level of evidence: B)

European Society of Cardiology and European Association for Cardio-Thoracic Surgery. ESC/EACTS Guidelines on Myocardial Revascularization, 2014.[3] (AGREE II Score: unavailable)

- For patients with moderate to severe CKD:
  ○ CABG should be considered over PCI in patients with multivessel CAD and symptoms/ischemia whose surgical risk profile is acceptable and life expectancy is beyond 1 year. (Recommendation class: IIa; Level of evidence: B)
  ○ PCI should be considered over CABG in patients with multivessel CAD and symptoms/ischemia whose surgical risk profile is high or life expectancy is less than 1 year. (Recommendation class: IIa; Level of evidence: B)
  ○ It should be considered to delay CABG after coronary angiography until the effect of contrast media on renal function has subsided. (Recommendation class: IIa; Level of evidence: B)
  ○ Off-pump CABG may be considered rather than on-pump CABG. (Recommendation class: IIa; Level of evidence: B)
  ○ New-generation drug-eluting stents are recommended over bare metal stents. (Recommendation class: I; Level of evidence: B)

Note: Additional recommendations for prevention of contrast-induced nephropathy in CKD patients are included in the complete guideline.

AUTHOR COMMENTARY

We searched the extant literature in PubMed and EMBASE, identifying the most recent high-quality systematic review and subsequent randomized, controlled trials (RCTs). We found 1 high-quality meta-analysis (AMSTAR [A Measurement Tool to Assess Systematic Reviews] Score = 79%) covering published observational studies through June 2010. Our overall search covered through April 2015.

Low-quality data suggest that both short- and long-term mortality in patients with ACS and comorbid renal disease are better in those who undergo revascularization than in those who receive only pharmacologic treatment (see **Table 1**). Although there was significant heterogeneity in the included studies, the results were consistent across studies and GFRs.

The evidence is low quality, primarily owing to the dearth of direct evidence of efficacy or harms of revascularization in the CKD population.[4,5] Although 40% of all patients presenting with ACS have some degree of renal impairment, those with CKD are commonly excluded from RCTs of revascularization procedures, resulting in study subjects who are likely to be healthier than patients seen in clinical practice. Additional methodological weaknesses include interventions that defy blinding and the potential for misclassification of acute kidney injury for CKD.[6] In addition, because of potential differences in GFR strata distributions, we were unable to calculate GFR–interval outcome rates and therefore report results anchored at zero.

In relation to harms, because of the underrepresentation of patients with CKD, RCTs of revascularization underestimate the frequency of bleeding.[7] The absolute increase in mortality caused by major bleeding in ACS is estimated to be 11% (95% confidence interval [CI], 8–14), with a number needed to harm of 9 (95% CI, 7–13).[7] Moreover, the incidence of periprocedural complications such as death, myocardial infarction, stroke, infection, and renal failure is increased in patients with CKD compared with those without renal dysfunction.[2]

The risk for developing *de novo* CAD, adverse outcomes, or death after an initial myocardial infarction increases markedly with decreases in GFR. This increased risk suggests that patients with CKD could benefit even more from an invasive strategy than patients without CKD.[8] In a UK registry study, CKD was present in 43.7% of all patients with non–ST-elevation ACS. After adjusting for covariables, revascularization was associated with a 30% reduction in 1-year mortality compared with medical management after coronary angiography (adjusted odds ratio, 0.66; 95% CI, 0.57–0.77), regardless of renal dysfunction severity. Early revascularization may thus offer similar survival benefit in patients with renal dysfunction.

The guidelines do not directly address the clinical question this report addresses.

GLOSSARY

ACS, acute coronary syndrome; AGREE II, Appraisal of Guidelines for Research and Evaluation; CABG, coronary artery bypass graft; CAD, coronary artery disease; CI, confidence interval; CKD, chronic kidney disease; GFR, glomerular filtration rate; GRADE, Grading of Recommendations Assessment, Development and Evaluation; NNT, number needed to treat; PCI, percutaneous coronary intervention; RCT, randomized controlled trial.

RECOMMENDED CITATION

Lascher S, Goldmann DR; Elsevier Evidence-Based Medicine Center: Evidence Review: Coronary Artery Revascularization in Patients with Acute Coronary Syndrome and Comorbid Renal Disease. Cardiol Clin 2016;34(4).

DISCLAIMER

Knowledge and best practice in this field are constantly changing. As new research and experience broaden our understanding, changes in research methods, professional practices, or medical treatment may become necessary.

Practitioners and researchers must always rely on their own experience and knowledge in evaluating and using any information, methods, compounds, or experiments described herein. In using such information or methods they should be mindful of their own safety and the safety of others, including parties for whom they have a professional responsibility.

To the fullest extent of the law, neither the Publisher nor the authors, contributors, or editors, assume any liability for any injury and/or damage to persons or property as a matter of products liability, negligence or otherwise, or from any use or operation of any methods, products, instructions, or ideas contained in the material herein.

Copyright © 2016 Elsevier Inc. All rights reserved.

REFERENCES

1. Huang HD, Alam M, Hamzeh I, et al. Patients with severe chronic kidney disease benefit from early revascularization after acute coronary syndrome. Int J Cardiol 2013;168(4):3741–6.
2. Levine GN, Bates ER, Blankenship JC, et al. 2011 ACCF/AHA/SCAI guideline for percutaneous coronary intervention. A report of the American College of Cardiology Foundation/American Heart Association Task Force on practice guidelines and the Society for Cardiovascular Angiography and Interventions. J Am Coll Cardiol 2011;58(24):e44–122.
3. Windecker S, Kolh P, Alfonso F, et al. ESC/EACTS Guidelines on myocardial revascularization. Eur Heart J 2014; 35(37):2541–619.
4. Seddon M, Curzen N. Coronary revascularisation in chronic kidney disease. Part II: acute coronary syndromes. J Ren Care 2010;36(Suppl 1):118–26.
5. Hanna EB, Chen AY, Roe MT, et al. Characteristics and in-hospital outcomes of patients with non-ST-segment elevation myocardial infarction and chronic kidney disease undergoing percutaneous coronary intervention. JACC Cardiovasc Interv 2011;4(9):1002–8.
6. Baber U, Stone GW, Weisz G, et al. Coronary plaque composition, morphology, and outcomes in patients with and without chronic kidney disease presenting with acute coronary syndromes. JACC Cardiovasc Imaging 2012; 5(Suppl 3):S53–61.
7. Steg PG, Huber K, Andreotti F, et al. Bleeding in acute coronary syndromes and percutaneous coronary interventions: position paper by the Working Group on Thrombosis of the European Society of Cardiology. Eur Heart J 2011; 32(15):1854–64.
8. Charytan DM, Wallentin L, Lagerqvist B, et al. Early angiography in patients with chronic kidney disease: a collaborative systematic review. Clin J Am Soc Nephrol 2009;4(6):1032–43.

Quick Evidence Synopsis
Percutaneous Coronary Intervention or Coronary Artery Bypass Grafting for Patients with Coronary Artery Disease

Date completed: October 16, 2015

EBM center contributors: Megan Sands-Lincoln, PhD, MPH and David R. Goldmann, MD

Clinical question: What are the benefits and harms of percutaneous coronary intervention (PCI) versus coronary artery bypass grafting (CABG) for multi-vessel, left main, and single-vessel proximal left anterior descending (LAD) coronary artery disease (CAD)?

What does the evidence conclude?

Intervention	Quality of Evidence	Balance Between Benefits and Harms
CABG vs PCI	Moderate	Trade-off between benefits and harms for both CABG and PCI, with CABG offering a mortality benefit over PCI in patients with multi-vessel CAD, especially those with significant risk factors, such as diabetes mellitus; the relative benefit of 1 procedure over another in reducing mortality is less clear in patients with less complex anatomic lesions. PCI offers some advantage in lower incidence of complicating stroke but a higher rate of need for subsequent target lesion reintervention compared with CABG.

Quality of evidence: Quality of evidence scale (Grading of Recommendations Assessment, Development and Evaluation [GRADE]): high, moderate, low, and very low. For more information on the GRADE rating system, see http://www.grade-workinggroup.org/index.htm.

Balance between benefits and harms: The Guideline Elements Model: beneficial, likely to be beneficial, unknown effectiveness, trade-off between benefits and harms, likely harmful, and harmful. For more information, see http://gem.med.yale.edu/default.htm.

What are the parameters of the authors' evidence search?

Population: adults with CAD, including multi-vessel (2- or 3-vessel disease; multi-vessel disease [MVD]), left main disease (LMD), or single-vessel proximal LAD, with or without diabetes

Setting: inpatient

Intervention: PCI

Comparator: CABG

Outcomes: mortality (all-cause); stroke; myocardial infarction; stent thrombosis (definite or probable stent thrombosis, time to occurrence); angiographic restenosis; and need for repeat revascularization

What is the basis for the conclusion?

Population: adults with CAD, including MVD (2 or 3 vessel), LMD, or single-vessel proximal LAD disease, with or without diabetes
Settings: inpatient
Intervention: PCI (bare-metal stents and drug-eluting stents)
Comparator: CABG (Table 1)

Cardiol Clin 34 (2016) 615–621
http://dx.doi.org/10.1016/j.ccl.2016.08.002
0733-8651/16

Table 1
Summary of recent systematic reviews addressing percutaneous coronary intervention versus coronary artery bypass grafting in patients with and without diabetes

Author (Year)	Study Type (Number of Participants)	Population, Intervention	Outcomes	Estimate of Effect (95% CI)	Key Results
Sipahi et al,[1] 2014	MA of 6 RCTs[a] (N = 6055)	Patients with MVD randomly assigned to CABG vs PCI (including both BMS and drug-eluting stent) 2 RCTs = 100% diabetic patients 4 RCTs = 33% diabetic patients[a] Included patients with stable and unstable angina	All-cause mortality, myocardial infarction, repeat revascularization, stroke, MACCE[a]	Mortality (all-cause): RR, 0.73 (95% CI, 0.62–0.86; P<.001) Stroke: RR, 1.36 (95% CI, 0.99–1.86; P<.06)	CABG favors lower risk of mortality. PCI may favor lower risk of stroke. Subanalysis demonstrated no difference in mortality outcome in participants with or without diabetes.
Smit et al,[2] 2015	MA of 31 RCTs (N = 15,004)	Patients with MVD, SVD, LAD, or LMD, with or without unstable angina randomly assigned to PCI (BMS and drug-eluting stents) vs CABG	All-cause mortality, myocardial infarction, repeat revascularization, stroke	Mortality (all-cause): OR, 1.1 (95% CI, 1.0–1.3); P = .05) Stroke: OR, 0.7 (0.5–0.9; P = .01)	All patient groups CABG favors lower risk of mortality. PCI favors lower risk of stroke.
Deb et al,[3] 2013	Systematic review[b] of 13 RCTs, 5 MAs LMD, N = 705 MVD, N = 1088[4]	Patients with MVD, LMD, or left ventricular dysfunction randomly assigned to CABG vs PCI (BMS and drug-eluting stents)	MACCE, stroke, mortality, repeat revascularization, myocardial infarction	*LMD* CABG vs PCI Mortality: RR, 0.88 (95% CI 0.58, 1.32) Stroke: 0.33 (95% CI 0.12, 0.92)[5] *MVD*[4] Mortality (all-cause): 11.4% vs 13.9% (P = .10) Stroke: 3.7% vs 2.4% (P = .09)	*LMD* There was no difference in mortality. PCI favors lower risk of stroke. *MVD* There was no difference in mortality or stroke outcomes.

Study	MA	Patients	Outcomes	Results	Overall
Al Ali,[6] 2014	MA of 7 RCTs (N = 5835)	Patients with MVD, LAD, or LMD randomly assigned to CABG vs PCI (drug-eluting stents) 48% of patients with diabetes	Mortality, stroke, myocardial infarction, revascularization	*Overall* Mortality: RR, 0.85 (95% CI 0.64, 1.12); Stroke: RR, 1.79 (95% CI 1.23, 2.62); *MVD* Mortality: RR, 0.73, (95% CI 0.56, 0.96); Stroke: RR: 1.72 (95% CI 1.02, 2.90); *LMD* Mortality: RR, 1.08 (95% CI 0.75, 1.57); Stroke: RR, 2.89 (95% CI 1.15, 7.27); *LAD* Mortality: RR, 2.34 (95% CI 0.64, 1.12); Stroke: RR, 5.07 (95% CI 0.21, 122.80).	*Overall* CABG favors reduced mortality. PCI favors reduced stroke. *MVD* CABG favors lower risk of mortality. PCI favors lower risk of stroke. *LMD* There was no difference in mortality. PCI favors lower risk of stroke. *LAD* There was no difference in mortality or stroke, but the effect estimate was unstable because of inadequate power.
Fanari et al,[7] 2014	MA of 6 RCTs (N = 5123)	Patients with MVD randomly assigned to CABG vs PCI with mostly drug-eluting stents; 60.5%–75.5% diabetes	All-cause mortality, stroke, myocardial infarction, target vessel revascularization	Mortality at 5 y: RR, 1.3 (95% CI 1.10, 1.54); Stroke: RR, 0.6 (95% CI 0.42, 0.86).	CABG favors reduced mortality. PCI favors reduced stroke.
Palmerini et al,[8] 2012	MA of 19 RCTs (N = 10,944) 12 RCTs (N = 7052)	Patients with MVD, SVD, or LMD with CAD randomly assigned to CABG and PCI	Stroke	Stroke at 30 d: OR, 2.94 [95% CI 1.69, 5.09]; Stroke at 12.1 mo subanalysis (N = 7052): 1.67 (95% CI 1.09, 2.56).	All patient groups Mortality outcome was NR. PCI favors reduced stroke.

Abbreviations: BMS, bare-metal stent; CI, confidence interval; LAD, single-vessel proximal left anterior descending; LMD, left main disease; MA, meta-analysis; MACCE, major adverse cardiovascular and cerebrovascular events (all-cause mortality, myocardial infarction, stroke, or repeat revascularization); NR, not reported; OR, odds ratio; RCT, randomized controlled trial; RR, relative risk; SR, systematic review; SVD, single-vessel disease.

[a] See Table 1 in the meta-analysis itself for addition information on median follow-up times and outcomes of interest stratified by trial and Table 2 in the article for information on the distribution of patient characteristics in the trials.

[b] This systematic review included 13 randomized controlled trials and 5 meta-analyses (MAs) but did not conduct an additional MA among the 13 included trials outlined in Table 2.[3]

What do clinical guidelines say?

National Institute for Health and Care Excellence. Management of Stable Angina. Last modified 2012.[9] (Appraisal of Guidelines for Research and Evaluation [AGREE] II score: unavailable)

- Consider revascularization (CABG or PCI) for people with stable angina whose symptoms are not satisfactorily controlled with optimal medical treatment.
- When either procedure would be appropriate, explain to patients the risks and benefits of PCI and CABG for people with anatomically less complex disease whose symptoms are not satisfactorily controlled with optimal medical treatment. If patients do not express a preference, take account of the evidence that suggests that PCI may be the more cost-effective procedure in selecting the course of treatment.
- When either procedure would be appropriate, take into account the potential survival advantage of CABG over PCI for people with MVD whose symptoms are not satisfactorily controlled with optimal medical treatment and who have diabetes, are more than 65 years old, or have anatomically complex 3-vessel disease, with or without involvement of the left main stem.
- Consider the relative risks and benefits of CABG and PCI for people with stable angina using a systematic approach to assess the severity and complexity of their coronary disease, in addition to other relevant clinical factors and comorbidities.

ACCF/AHA Guideline for Coronary Artery Bypass Graft Surgery: A Report of the American College of Cardiology Foundation/American Heart Association Task Force on Practice Guidelines[10] **and ACCF/AHA/SCAI Guideline for Percutaneous Coronary Intervention: A Report of the American College of Cardiology Foundation/American Heart Association Task Force on Practice Guidelines and the Society for Cardiovascular Angiography and Interventions, 2011.**[11] (AGREE II score: 73%)

Recommendations for revascularization to improve survival (class I[a])

- Left main CAD revascularization: CABG to improve survival is recommended for patients with significant (>50% diameter stenosis) left main coronary artery stenosis. (Level of evidence: B)
- Non–left main CAD revascularization: CABG to improve survival is beneficial in patients with significant (>70% diameter) stenosis in 3 major coronary arteries (with or without involvement of the proximal LAD artery) or in the proximal LAD artery plus 1 other major coronary artery. (Level of evidence: B)

Recommendations for revascularization to improve symptoms (class I[a])

- CABG or PCI to improve symptoms is beneficial in patients with 1 or more significant (>70% diameter) coronary artery stenoses amenable to revascularization and unacceptable angina despite guideline-directed medical therapy. (Level of evidence: A)

Recommendations regarding patient risk factors

- It is important to consider patient characteristics and consult with both an interventional cardiologist and a cardiac surgeon to decide on optimal revascularization strategy, especially with critically ill patients. Clinical characteristics to consider include coexisting diabetes mellitus and/or chronic kidney disease status, completeness of revascularization possible, left ventricular systolic dysfunction, unstable angina/non-ST segment elevation myocardial infarction, and previous CABG.

Level of evidence A: multiple populations evaluated, data derived from multiple randomized controlled trials (RCTs) or meta-analyses

Level of evidence B: Limited populations evaluated, data derived from a single RCT or nonrandomized study

Level of evidence C: Very limited populations evaluated, only consensus opinion of experts, case studies, or standards of care

---

[a]Class I defined as follows: benefit outweighs the risk, and the procedure/treatment SHOULD be performed/administered.

AUTHOR COMMENTARY

Consideration of coronary artery revascularization is indicated in patients with symptomatic but stable coronary artery disease in whom medical therapy has proven insufficient and in those with acute coronary syndrome. As such, there is a large body of literature comparing the benefits and harms of coronary artery bypass surgery to PCI in a spectrum of patients with CAD.

The authors searched PubMed, EMBASE, the Cochrane Database of Systematic Reviews, and the National Guideline Clearinghouse for systematic reviews, meta-analyses, RCTs, and guidelines on trials of CABG versus PCI in patients with CAD. The authors retrieved 3 relevant guidelines[9–11] and 6 pertinent systematic reviews and meta-analyses.[1–3,6–8] For the purposes of this evidence review, the authors excluded the primary RCTs retrieved in the search, focusing only on the reviews and meta-analyses, and also excluded any studies focusing on patients with diabetes,[12–22] renal disease, or the very elderly.[23–28] Outcomes for mortality and stroke are presented in **Table 1**.

In comparing PCI and CABG in patients included in these studies, the major overarching findings indicate decreased risk of all-cause mortality among patients undergoing CABG versus PCI at the cost of increased risk of stroke in those undergoing CABG. However, given that this is a broad overview of key findings, the authors did not elaborate on additional specific patient considerations that would be included in decision-making, including the presence of chronic kidney disease, specifics of coronary artery anatomy, lesion complexity, cardiac function, or other comorbid conditions.

It has been suggested that scoring algorithms, including the synergy between PCI with taxus and cardiac surgery (SYNTAX) score for determining the complexity of the underlying lesions, may be useful in determining the relative appropriateness and safety of PCI and CABG. The SYNTAX score is an angiographic grading tool that combines several other classification systems and expert opinion and can be a useful tool in identifying patients who are appropriate for one or the other. More recently, an enhanced SYNTAX II score was developed with the intent of improving its sensitivity.[29] Other measures that account for patient comorbidities, including the Charlson Comorbidity Index and EuroSCORE, may be useful in determining the treatment course. Although evidence indicates the potential value in these scoring algorithms specifically in subpopulations with renal insufficiency and CAD,[23–27] additional prospective studies evaluating their clinical utility are needed.

Current clinical practice guidelines recommend CABG over PCI for patients with diabetes and MVD. The evidence is less clear for patients with LMD and single-vessel proximal left anterior disease in patients without diabetes or with other comorbidities. Although not fully discussed in this evidence review, it is important to consider observed sex differences in outcomes, with higher rates of in-hospital mortality among women undergoing CABG and higher rates of subsequent revascularization among women undergoing PCI.[30] Other considerations include local and regional resources and the expertise and experience of individual practitioners.

GLOSSARY

AGREE II, Appraisal of Guidelines for Research and Evaluation; BMS, bare-metal stent; CABG, coronary artery bypass grafting; CAD, coronary artery disease; CI, confidence interval; GRADE, Grading of Recommendations Assessment, Development and Evaluation; LAD, single-vessel proximal left anterior disease; LMD, left main disease; MA, meta-analysis; MACCE, major adverse cardiovascular and cerebrovascular events; MVD, multi-vessel disease; NNT, number needed to treat; NR, not reported; OR, odds ratio; PCI, percutaneous coronary intervention; RCT, randomized controlled trial; RR, relative risk; SR, systematic review; SVD, single-vessel disease.

RECOMMENDED CITATION

Sands-Lincoln M, Goldmann DR. Elsevier Evidence-Based Medicine Center: Evidence Review: Percutaneous Coronary Intervention or Coronary Artery Bypass Grafting for Patients With Coronary Artery Disease. Cardiol Clin 2016;34(4).

DISCLAIMER

Knowledge and best practice in this field are constantly changing. As new research and experience broaden our understanding, changes in research methods, professional practices, or medical treatment may become necessary.

Practitioners and researchers must always rely on their own experience and knowledge in evaluating and using any information, methods, compounds, or experiments described herein. In using such information or methods they should be mindful of their own safety and the safety of others, including parties for whom they have a professional responsibility.

To the fullest extent of the law, neither the publisher nor the authors, contributors, or editors assume any liability for any injury and/or damage to persons or property as a matter of products liability, negligence or otherwise, or from any use or operation of any methods, products, instructions, or ideas contained in the material herein.

Copyright © 2016 Elsevier Inc. All rights reserved.

REFERENCES

1. Sipahi I, Akay MH, Dagdelen S, et al. Coronary artery bypass grafting vs percutaneous coronary intervention and long-term mortality and morbidity in multivessel disease: meta-analysis of randomized clinical trials of the arterial grafting and stenting era. JAMA Intern Med 2014;174(2):223–30.

2. Smit Y, Vlayen J, Koppenaal H, et al. Percutaneous coronary intervention versus coronary artery bypass grafting: a meta-analysis. J Thorac Cardiovasc Surg 2015;149(3):831–8.e1-3.

3. Deb S, Wijeysundera HC, Ko DT, et al. Coronary artery bypass graft surgery vs percutaneous interventions in coronary revascularization: a systematic review. JAMA 2013;310(19):2086–95.

4. Mohr FW, Morice MC, Kappetein AP, et al. Coronary artery bypass graft surgery versus percutaneous coronary intervention in patients with three-vessel disease and left main coronary disease: 5-year follow-up of the randomised, clinical SYNTAX trial. Lancet (Lond) 2013;381(9867):629–38.

5. Morice MC, Serruys PW, Kappetein AP, et al. Five-year outcomes in patients with left main disease treated with either percutaneous coronary intervention or coronary artery bypass grafting in the synergy between percutaneous coronary intervention with taxus and cardiac surgery trial. Circulation 2014;129(23):2388–94.

6. Al Ali J, Franck C, Filion KB, et al. Coronary artery bypass graft surgery versus percutaneous coronary intervention with first-generation drug-eluting stents: a meta-analysis of randomized controlled trials. JACC Cardiovasc Interv 2014;7(5):497–506.

7. Fanari Z, Weiss SA, Zhang W, et al. Short, intermediate and long term outcomes of CABG vs. PCI with DES in patients with multivessel coronary artery disease. Meta-analysis of six randomized controlled trials. Eur J Cardiovasc Med 2014;3(1):382–9.

8. Palmerini T, Biondi-Zoccai G, Reggiani LB, et al. Risk of stroke with coronary artery bypass graft surgery compared with percutaneous coronary intervention. J Am Coll Cardiol 2012;60(9):798–805.

9. National Clinical Guideline Centre, National Institute for Health and Clinical Excellence. Management of stable angina. 2011. Available at: http://www.guideline.gov/content.aspx?id=34825&search=stable+angina. Accessed September 21, 2015.

10. Hillis LD, Smith PK, Anderson JL, et al. 2011 ACCF/AHA guideline for coronary artery bypass graft surgery: a report of the American College of Cardiology Foundation/American Heart Association Task Force on Practice Guidelines. Circulation 2011;124(23):e652–735.

11. Levine GN, Bates ER, Blankenship JC, et al. 2011 ACCF/AHA/SCAI guideline for percutaneous coronary intervention: a report of the American College of Cardiology Foundation/American Heart Association Task Force on Practice Guidelines and the Society for Cardiovascular Angiography and Interventions. Circulation 2011; 124(23):e574–651.

12. Ariyaratne TV, Ademi Z, Yap CH, et al. Prolonged effectiveness of coronary artery bypass surgery versus drug-eluting stents in diabetics with multi-vessel disease: an updated systematic review and meta-analysis. Int J Cardiol 2014;176(2):346–53.

13. De Luca G, Schaffer A, Verdoia M, et al. Meta-analysis of 14 trials comparing bypass grafting vs drug-eluting stents in diabetic patients with multivessel coronary artery disease. Nutr Metab Cardiovasc Dis 2014;24(4):344–54.

14. Fanari Z, Weiss SA, Weintraub WS. Comparative effectiveness of revascularization strategies in stable ischemic heart disease: current perspective and literature review. Expert Rev Cardiovasc Ther 2013;11(10):1321–36.

15. Gao F, Zhou YJ, Shen H, et al. Meta-analysis of percutaneous coronary intervention versus coronary artery bypass graft surgery in patients with diabetes and left main and/or multivessel coronary artery disease. Acta Diabetol 2013;50(5):765–73.

16. Hakeem A, Garg N, Bhatti S, et al. Effectiveness of percutaneous coronary intervention with drug-eluting stents compared with bypass surgery in diabetics with multivessel coronary disease: comprehensive systematic review and meta-analysis of randomized clinical data. J Am Heart Assoc 2013;2(4):e000354.

17. Huang F, Lai W, Chan C, et al. Comparison of bypass surgery and drug-eluting stenting in diabetic patients with left main and/or multivessel disease: a systematic review and meta-analysis of randomized and nonrandomized studies. Cardiol J 2015;22(2):123–34.
18. Li R, Yang S, Tang L, et al. Meta-analysis of the effect of percutaneous coronary intervention on chronic total coronary occlusions. J Card Surg 2014;9:41.
19. Tu B, Rich B, Labos C, et al. Coronary revascularization in diabetic patients: a systematic review and Bayesian network meta-analysis. Ann Intern Med 2014;161(10):724–32.
20. Verma S, Farkouh ME, Yanagawa B, et al. Comparison of coronary artery bypass surgery and percutaneous coronary intervention in patients with diabetes: a meta-analysis of randomised controlled trials. Lancet Diabetes Endocrinol 2013;1(4):317–28.
21. Zhang F, Yang Y, Hu D, et al. Percutaneous coronary intervention (PCI) versus coronary artery bypass grafting (CABG) in the treatment of diabetic patients with multi-vessel coronary disease: a meta-analysis. Diabetes Res Clin Pract 2012;97(2):178–84.
22. Andrés Jadue T, Roberto González L, Manuel JILL. Meta-analysis of coronary artery bypass surgery compared to percutaneous transluminal angioplasty with stent in diabetic patients. Rev Med Chil 2012;140(5):640–8.
23. Chang TI, Leong TK, Kazi DS, et al. Comparative effectiveness of coronary artery bypass grafting and percutaneous coronary intervention for multivessel coronary disease in a community-based population with chronic kidney disease. Am Heart J 2013;165(5):800–8, 808.e1-2.
24. Chang TI, Shilane D, Kazi DS, et al. Multivessel coronary artery bypass grafting versus percutaneous coronary intervention in ESRD. J Am Soc Nephrol 2012;23(12):2042–9.
25. Deo SV, Shah IK, Dunlay SM, et al. Coronary artery bypass grafting versus drug-eluting stents in patients with end-stage renal disease. J Card Surg 2014;29(2):163–9.
26. Domanski MJ, Farkouh ME, Zak V, et al. Predictors of stroke associated with coronary artery bypass grafting in patients with diabetes mellitus and multivessel coronary artery disease. Am J Cardiol 2015;115(10):1382–8.
27. Marui A, Kimura T, Nishiwaki N, et al. Percutaneous coronary intervention versus coronary artery bypass grafting in patients with end-stage renal disease requiring dialysis (5-year outcomes of the CREDO-Kyoto PCI/CABG Registry Cohort-2). Am J Cardiol 2014;114(4):555–61.
28. Nicolini F, Contini GA, Fortuna D, et al. Coronary artery surgery versus percutaneous coronary intervention in octogenarians: long-term results. Ann Thorac Surg 2015;99(2):567–74.
29. Farooq V, Vergouwe Y, Raber L, et al. Combined anatomical and clinical factors for the long-term risk stratification of patients undergoing percutaneous coronary intervention: the Logistic Clinical SYNTAX score. Eur Heart J 2012;33(24):3098–104.
30. D'Ascenzo F, Barbero U, Moretti C, et al. Percutaneous coronary intervention versus coronary artery bypass graft for stable angina: meta-regression of randomized trials. Contemp Clin Trials 2014;38(1):51–8.

Index

Note: Page numbers of article titles are in **boldface** type.

Cardiol Clin 34 (2016) 623–626
http://dx.doi.org/10.1016/S0733-8651(16)30091-1
0733-8651/16/$ – see front matter

UNITED STATES POSTAL SERVICE® Statement of Ownership, Management, and Circulation
(All Periodicals Publications Except Requester Publications)

1. Publication Title	CARDIOLOGY CLINICS
2. Publication Number	000 – 701
3. Filing Date	9/18/2016
4. Issue Frequency	FEB, MAY, AUG, NOV
5. Number of Issues Published Annually	4
6. Annual Subscription Price	$305.00

7. Complete Mailing Address of Known Office of Publication (Not printer) (Street, city, county, state, and ZIP+4®)

ELSEVIER INC.
360 PARK AVENUE SOUTH
NEW YORK, NY 10010-1710

Contact Person: STEPHEN R. BUSHING
Telephone (Include area code): 215-239-3688

8. Complete Mailing Address of Headquarters or General Business Office of Publisher (Not printer)

ELSEVIER INC.
360 PARK AVENUE SOUTH
NEW YORK, NY 10010-1710

9. Full Names and Complete Mailing Addresses of Publisher, Editor, and Managing Editor (Do not leave blank)

Publisher (Name and complete mailing address)

ADRIANNE BRIGIDO, ELSEVIER INC.
1600 JOHN F KENNEDY BLVD. SUITE 1800
PHILADELPHIA, PA 19103-2899

Editor (Name and complete mailing address)

LAUREN ELISE BOYLE, ELSEVIER INC.
1600 JOHN F KENNEDY BLVD. SUITE 1800
PHILADELPHIA, PA 19103-2899

Managing Editor (Name and complete mailing address)

PATRICK MANLEY, ELSEVIER INC.
1600 JOHN F KENNEDY BLVD. SUITE 1800
PHILADELPHIA, PA 19103-2899

10. Owner (Do not leave blank. If the publication is owned by a corporation, give the name and address of the corporation immediately followed by the names and addresses of all stockholders owning or holding 1 percent or more of the total amount of stock. If not owned by a corporation, give the names and addresses of the individual owners. If owned by a partnership or other unincorporated firm, give its name and address as well as those of each individual owner. If the publication is published by a nonprofit organization, give its name and address.)

Full Name	Complete Mailing Address
WHOLLY OWNED SUBSIDIARY OF REED/ELSEVIER, US HOLDINGS	1600 JOHN F KENNEDY BLVD. SUITE 1800 PHILADELPHIA, PA 19103-2899

11. Known Bondholders, Mortgagees, and Other Security Holders Owning or Holding 1 Percent or More of Total Amount of Bonds, Mortgages, or Other Securities. If none, check box ▶ ☐ None

Full Name	Complete Mailing Address
N/A	

12. Tax Status (For completion by nonprofit organizations authorized to mail at nonprofit rates) (Check one)
The purpose, function, and nonprofit status of this organization and the exempt status for federal income tax purposes:
☐ Has Not Changed During Preceding 12 Months
☐ Has Changed During Preceding 12 Months (Publisher must submit explanation of change with this statement)

13. Publication Title	14. Issue Date for Circulation Data Below
CARDIOLOGY CLINICS	AUGUST 2016

15. Extent and Nature of Circulation		Average No. Copies Each Issue During Preceding 12 Months	No. Copies of Single Issue Published Nearest to Filing Date
a. Total Number of Copies (Net press run)		372	411
b. Paid Circulation (By Mail and Outside the Mail)	(1) Mailed Outside-County Paid Subscriptions Stated on PS Form 3541 (include paid distribution above nominal rate, advertiser's proof copies, and exchange copies)	143	177
	(2) Mailed In-County Paid Subscriptions Stated on PS Form 3541 (include paid distribution above nominal rate, advertiser's proof copies, and exchange copies)	0	0
	(3) Paid Distribution Outside the Mails Including Sales Through Dealers and Carriers, Street Vendors, Counter Sales, and Other Paid Distribution Outside USPS®	72	94
	(4) Paid Distribution by Other Classes of Mail Through the USPS (e.g. First-Class Mail®)	0	0
c. Total Paid Distribution (Sum of 15b (1), (2), (3), and (4))		215	271
d. Free or Nominal Rate Distribution (By Mail and Outside the Mail)	(1) Free or Nominal Rate Outside-County Copies included on PS Form 3541	20	40
	(2) Free or Nominal Rate In-County Copies included on PS Form 3541	0	0
	(3) Free or Nominal Rate Copies Mailed at Other Classes Through the USPS (e.g. First-Class Mail)	0	0
	(4) Free or Nominal Rate Distribution Outside the Mail (Carriers or other means)	0	0
e. Total Free or Nominal Rate Distribution (Sum of 15d (1), (2), (3) and (4))		20	40
f. Total Distribution (Sum of 15c and 15e)		235	311
g. Copies not Distributed (See Instructions to Publishers #4 (page #3))		137	100
h. Total (Sum of 15f and g)		372	411
i. Percent Paid (15c divided by 15f times 100)		94%	87%

* If you are claiming electronic copies, go to line 16 on page 3. If you are not claiming electronic copies, skip to line 17 on page 3.

16. Electronic Copy Circulation	Average No. Copies Each Issue During Preceding 12 Months	No. Copies of Single Issue Published Nearest to Filing Date
a. Paid Electronic Copies ▶	0	0
b. Total Paid Print Copies (Line 15c) + Paid Electronic Copies (Line 16a) ▶	215	271
c. Total Print Distribution (Line 15f) + Paid Electronic Copies (Line 16a) ▶	235	311
d. Percent Paid (Both Print & Electronic Copies) (16b divided by 16c × 100) ▶	94%	87%

☒ I certify that 50% of all my distributed copies (electronic and print) are paid above a nominal price.

17. Publication of Statement of Ownership
☒ If the publication is a general publication, publication of this statement is required. Will be printed in the NOVEMBER 2016 issue of this publication. ☐ Publication not required.

18. Signature and Title of Editor, Publisher, Business Manager, or Owner

STEPHEN R. BUSHING - INVENTORY DISTRIBUTION CONTROL MANAGER

Date: 9/18/2016

I certify that all information furnished on this form is true and complete. I understand that anyone who furnishes false or misleading information on this form or who omits material or information requested on the form may be subject to criminal sanctions (including fines and imprisonment) and/or civil sanctions (including civil penalties).

PS Form **3526**, July 2014 (Page 1 of 4 (see instructions page 4)) PSN: 7530-01-000-9931 PRIVACY NOTICE: See our privacy policy on www.usps.com.

PS Form **3526**, July 2014 (Page 2 of 4)

PS Form **3526**, July 2014 (Page 3 of 4)

PRIVACY NOTICE: See our privacy policy on www.usps.com.

Moving?

Make sure your subscription moves with you!

To notify us of your new address, find your **Clinics Account Number** (located on your mailing label above your name), and contact customer service at:

Email: journalscustomerservice-usa@elsevier.com

800-654-2452 (subscribers in the U.S. & Canada)
314-447-8871 (subscribers outside of the U.S. & Canada)

Fax number: 314-447-8029

**Elsevier Health Sciences Division
Subscription Customer Service
3251 Riverport Lane
Maryland Heights, MO 63043**

*To ensure uninterrupted delivery of your subscription, please notify us at least 4 weeks in advance of move.

Printed and bound by CPI Group (UK) Ltd, Croydon, CR0 4YY

03/10/2024

01040298-0003